KIDS IN CRISIS

(Book 2)

–PICU Kids, Our Heroes

Tabitha B. C. Abel

KIDS IN CRISIS –PICU Kids, Our Heroes
Book 2

First Printing, 2019
ISBN: 978-1-6990-5663-9

Cover Design by Fiverr.com/ultrakhan22

Weekly Blog Tabel Talk@TabithaBCAbel
www.TabithaAbel.webs.com

DEDICATION

To PICU healthcare professionals
who care for critically ill children.
God bless you.

Kids can break our hearts,
but PICU Kids are still Our Heroes
—and God's children

ENDORSEMENTS

Ronald M. Perkin, MD
Professor and Chair, Emeritus

*Department of Pediatrics, Brody School of Medicine,
East Carolina University, Greenville, North Carolina*

*Former Medical Director, PICU (1988-2000) Loma Linda
University Children's Hospital, Loma Linda, California*

*I have been involved in the practice of Medicine for over forty
years. For thirty-four of those years, I took care of critically ill and
injured children. In my opinion, the PICU is the heart of a Children's
Hospital. A TEAM of individuals is responsible for the care given to
the acutely ill or injured child: physicians, nurses, respiratory care
practitioners, pediatric-specialist pharmacists, and child-life
professionals, to name a few. The cornerstone of these is the nursing
staff; the PICU is only as good as its nursing staff.*

Caring for these children is a real calling. Emotions are high when dealing with children who are suddenly fighting for their lives. Many of the children were previously well and filled with potential but now, if they survive, may face life as differently-abled individuals. The children are not the only ones affected: parents, the extended family, and the medical team are also impacted. Even now, there are not many nights that I do not dream about caring for these critically ill children. I find it difficult to speak with people about my experiences unless they are familiar with the PICU. I cannot find the words to express the full range of emotions —not to mention the absolute horror of some of the cases.

Tabitha Abel has given us, the PICU TEAM/Community, a voice. Most importantly, Tabitha's voice is the voice of a seasoned PICU nurse, a TEAM member who spent 12-hour (and many times longer) shifts at the bedside of these critically ill and injured patients. A person who experienced the full gambit of emotions from the patient, the parents, the family, and from other TEAM members. Do yourself a favor and read the stories that Tabitha has written for you. Experience the life of the PICU through the eyes of a veteran PICU nurse who is also a mother. Feel the joy, sadness, suffering, and pain that a day in the PICU brings. I promise you will not need the made-for-television-stories about a "Medical Center." If you a pay close attention, you may even sense the presence of God.

* * *

Ann Altaffer, MSN, RN

Retired Charge Nurse in Two Large, Metropolitan PICUs

Emotions run high in the PICU. Children are not expected to suddenly become critically ill. Tabitha captures those emotions in **KIDS IN CRISIS –PICU Kids, Our Heroes** *from the perspective of the patient, the family and the staff. Readers will feel the conflicting emotions a PICU nurse feels each shift.*

* * *

Katherine Dalke, MSN, RN, Nurse Manager

Pediatric Intensive Care Unit (1979-2001)
Loma Linda University Children's Hospital

The KIDS IN CRISIS trilogy is a no-holds-barred peek into the life of a Registered Nurse working in one of the most stressful, challenging, heart-wrenching areas of a hospital – the Pediatric Intensive Care Unit. Abel's incisive writing style reveals the complexity and compassion of the environment with her occasional irreverent humor. Her unique perspective provides the reader with a clear understanding of life in the PICU and how she and her colleagues survived and saved the lives of countless children. Abel's dedication to her work shines through in KIDS IN CRISIS –PICU Kids, Our Heroes.

ACKNOWLEDGEMENTS

KIDS IN CRISIS: PICU Kids, Our Heroes is the second book in the KIDS IN CRISIS trilogy. PICU Kids are quintessential to this book being written, and my special thanks goes to the many kids whose stories do not appear in this memoir. They are the "meat and potatoes" of a PICU nurse's life and no doubt, the apple of their parents' eyes. And yet these hundreds of kids, don't get a mention and are lost in the mists of time, leaving us with Our Heroes of this memoir. Thank you.

I have worked among an amazingly talented, hard-working and diverse group of colleagues who are focused on our young patients, Our Heroes. Thank you for working with me, helping me through rough times, encouraging me and laughing with me. With this second book, my special thanks goes to two friends who were my line editors. Thank you. You made me look better than I am!

KIDS IN CRISIS: PICU Kids, Our Heroes is endorsed by Dr. Ronald M. Perkin who has dedicated his life to caring for critically ill children and passing on his knowledge to generations of pediatricians and pediatric intensivists. I had the honor of being part of his Team for a number of years. He was a Director who humbly denied that he knew everything about Our Kids —and yet he did. He made my day when he said he would like to endorse KIDS IN CRISIS. Thank you, Dr. Perkin. My thanks too to Katherine Dalke, a Nurse Manager who managed a huge staff with aplomb —but did not know everything that happened on her unit in her absence, and to Ann Altaffer, a long-time friend and colleague, who was an able, professional, kind, Charge Nurse who stood up for her staff and Our Kids.

My family still deserves a mention because they endured my long work hours and tolerated my wild ideas, and still do. Thank you, Todd Cooper and Yoon, Ross Cooper and Alyssa and my faithful daughter, Joelle Cooper, a Special Ed teacher who works diligently in a school district not too far from my alma mater.

My hope is that the stories will come to life as they are read and that readers will understand the joy and heartache those of us working with critically ill children experience in our work. I also want to tempt up-and-coming nurses and pediatricians to join us in this experience. My thanks too to EMS staff who drop off their little charges with us, trusting us to build on their good start. It is difficult to understand what a kid goes through in the PICU, but it takes a village to help some kids reach their potential after a stay with us. Thank you parents, health care providers, chaplains, law enforcement personnel, social workers and, teachers, coaches, encouragers, parents and spiritual guides who help them recover at home. Thank you for having a heart for children, for critically ill children, and for wanting to understand the Pediatric ICU better. It is a place where angels wait at bedsides and miracles happen, sometimes, praise God.

Tabitha B. C. Abel
DrPH, MSN, RN

TABLE OF CONTENTS

PREFACE

KIDS IN CRISIS is a series of three books about life in a pediatric ICU: children who are critically ill, their families and the medical personnel who provide care to our patients, especially the nurses. In the first book, *KIDS IN CRISIS —Pediatric ICU 101* readers met the staff and a few kids. Now they will meet more of Our Heroes, PICU Kids, and their families.

Each child and family have their own story to tell but the stories in *KIDS IN CRISIS —PICU Kids, Our Heroes* are real-life stories that have been adapted for this memoir, using different names and details, although the stories are based on specific occurrences in a number of locations. Some of the characters are an amalgam of people. However, Tabitha, the author and a PICU nurse, is the constant. She records the stories from the bedside through the lens of past childhood experiences and her present role as a Christian, parent and nurse. It all happens in Inland Valley Children's Hospital, a fictitious place with a large PICU and other pediatric floors.

Still to come is *KIDS IN CRISIS, Families in Crisis,* the final book in the trilogy which focuses more on our Heroes' families who endure a child's admission to the PICU filled with fear tempered with love and compassion –and also those families who unfortunately do not fall into this category.

*** *

You're braver than you believe,

and stronger than you seem,

and smarter than you think.

A.A. Milne/Christopher Robin

*** *

CHAPTER 1

PICU Kids et al.

I CAN'T SAY that I have a wonderful relationship with all my patients, because –I don't, and some shifts go better than others. Some are emotionally or physically draining (or both), or simply routine. It can be difficult when dealing with challenging families or complicated clinical situations, and yet, despite that, some shifts are uplifting and energizing. Shifts are much like life. They are not all happy-happy, joy-joy. But what matters most, is what we make of each shift –or our lives.

I had always wanted to be a nurse, at least that is what I thought was the case, until I realized that being a nurse was what my mother actually determined me to be. So that is what I became. That was when parents spoke, and kids did as they were told. For me, with absolutely no adult other than my mother to discuss this important matter with, I did as she said. It seemed to be good advice.

My family was atypical for the early 1960s because my parents divorced when I was very young. I was the only kid in my class who had divorced parents, unlike today. In a sad way, my nuclear family was ahead of the times! I was the last of five children and lived with my mother and the next child up in the family, Rebecca. Mum was in her forties when she had me, again, unheard of then. We lived in small villages and hamlets in southern England, always in the country, always away from shops and distractions. My other siblings, two full sisters, and a full brother, were much older than me. When I was relatively young, they left home, one at a time, to live abroad. My sisters to Greece and Australia, and my brother taught in Uganda for a while before going to live in America. Could they get any further away from us if they tried? And, without social media, my siblings could have been in outer space as far as I was concerned.

We had no distractions at home other than school work, our dogs, playing the piano, listening to the BBC on the radio and knitting. Life was slow. I still love playing the piano and can hold my own in church services, at weddings (with extra practice) and funerals. In my twenties, I decided that teaching the piano was not the career for me. I wasn't talented enough and I didn't practice enough. However, playing the piano still gives me great pleasure. and now, as a relatively inexperienced flautist, I enjoy the challenges of learning a wind instrument.

Our car disappeared when I was seven years old. One day, it wasn't there. I learned later that we did not have enough money to run it. With no transport other than our legs, we used the busses or hopped on our bicycles, thinking nothing of biking five miles somewhere, just because we needed to get there. The roller-skating rink was four miles away, so Rebecca and I biked there occasionally, and enjoyed the outing. The seaside was a little more than three miles from my home and an excursion took the whole afternoon. In our teens, my sister and I biked to the pebbly beach on a pathway across the marshes and over the London to North Kent high-speed railway line. We then biked the last mile to swim in the cold English Channel – and enjoyed it.

Despite there being rarely anyone else on the beach, we had no adult supervision. We had no thoughts of drowning —or being killed on the railway line. However, one day, when carrying my bike across the level crossing, AKA train-tracks, I turned to see a speeding train bearing down on me, blowing its horn. I was terrified. From then on, I checked the line more carefully. I had learned my lesson. Perhaps though, our youthful activities and enjoyment fed into my love of triathlons and road races that I still participate in today. With a can-do attitude that my mother expected of us, I set about making things happen if I wanted to do them.

There was no question that my sister Rebecca was academically brilliant, and would be a teacher, like our eldest sister —who was also smart. When I was bold enough to talk to my mother about what I should do with my life, her exact words were, "You're stupid enough to be a nurse, Tabitha." I unwisely thought she was right, and became a nurse like my second, "not-so-bright" sister, who was a competent surgical nurse working with the flying doctor in the outback in Western Australia. More importantly, this sister was also a very talented artist —which I wasn't.

With hindsight, being told "I was stupid enough" for anything, displayed my mother's critical, negative attitude.

She did not intentionally put me down, but as parents, I believe it is our job to encourage our children to be strong, resourceful, capable and fun-loving, so that they take on the world, and succeed. I eventually caught on and those characteristics fostered in me a determination to disprove her. Perhaps that is why it wasn't until I was forty, that I eventually completed a doctoral degree –which did not impress her one whit. Sadly, that same attitude contributed to my siblings moving far away from home.

So I learned to deal with the rough patches in life. I'd hang on, and tough it out. That worked for me, but was not always popular with my patient's parents, or my patients. I wanted to help them to "hang tough". To not give up. I knew that bad times didn't last forever, whether they were life-threatening illnesses, annoying parents, or lazy colleagues. And if it didn't work out? Pick up the pieces and move on. Every cloud eventually had a silver lining.

* * *

The rooms in the PedsICU are single patient rooms whether the kid is small enough to be comfortable in an infant warmer (which takes up less than three square feet), or big enough to need a regular, adult-sized bed, or even an oversized bed. The room also provides enough space for all the medical equipment a child might require, adequate space for a nurse to maneuver herself around the patient and equipment, extra space for personal items and for two visitors at the bedside, and then some.

Jaden was only 12-years-old when he spent more than six weeks in the PICU because a small nick on his knee turned septic. He was an incredible six-feet tall. He had first gone to an out-of-state ER for the problem. He had been sent home without antibiotic coverage, after all, it was only a small nick. The second visit had him staying in an out-lying hospital's ICU for a week, slowly getting worse and worse, until he was transported to our PICU, seriously ill and in danger of losing his leg, and possibly his life.

After a few surgeries treating raging, infected fasciitis, long, painful dressing changes and twice daily, hour-long, hyperbaric-oxygen treatments, this giant kid made it out of the PICU alive, to the Step-down ICU, and eventually to a basic pediatric unit.

Two months after his admission, Jaden walked (with a limp) from the door of the PedsICU, along the twenty-foot hallway, to the secretary's desk. "Is BJ here?" he asked.

BJ had been his Primary Nurse and cared for him throughout his six-week stay in PedsICU.

"She sure is," the secretary answered. "I'll get her for you. She'll be s-o-oo surprised to see you." She turned to the intercom. "Come on down BJ! You have a visitor!"

BJ, a lot shorter than Jaden's six-feet, broke into tears when she saw the giant waiting to see her. "I cannot believe it, Jaden. You look terrific," she said. It was a silver-lining moment for BJ. She gave Jaden a big hug as he squirmed, and Jaden's mom put her arm around BJ.

"We had to come and see you before we left, didn't we Jaden?" she said proudly looking up at her son. "Jaden is going home tomorrow."

BJ bent down and scrutinized Jaden's knee carefully. "That leg is great, Jaden," she said after the inspection.

"BJ, I want to thank you," Jaden said quietly.

"He really did want to thank you BJ," his mom interjected. "He insisted."

"You were the best nurse I ever had," Jaden said.

"Yes BJ," his mother added. "You gave us hope when we had none."

BJ was speechless with joy. She pointed heavenwards.

"Give Him the glory."

That type of experience is what makes a PICU nurse's day —being sought out, and thanked. Those silver-lining moments are serendipitous and delightful.

* * *

Simon was a regular kid who had been bitten by a rattlesnake, on his ankle. The California Desert has many rattlers that, when disturbed, will strike out at a person who troubles them, and some kids tease rattlesnakes even though desert dwellers know full-well that they should respect them. Simon was 11-years-old, and the snake had bitten, twice, on his right ankle. First, he was transported by paramedics to a small, local ER, and then flown by the Transport Team from the outlying hospital to our PICU, where I became his nurse. His worried family arrived shortly after he was admitted. Understandably, they were very concerned about his condition and the possibility that he would not pull through.

As Inland Valley Children's Hospital is near the high desert, our PICU occasionally received snake-bite kids. For the first two nights of his stay Simon was sedated, and on the ventilator. His was a one-to-one list, the type that was mildly challenging, but never out of control. We gave him anti-venom IV, and when destabilizing complications arose, they were treated. By the third full day, he was ready to be extubated.

As I was then off duty, Kai became his nurse for the next two nights. When I returned to work, I had to take another list. During a lull in caring for my new patients, I stopped by Simon's room to chat with Kai. Simon was almost asleep.

"How's Simon doing Kai?" I asked. "When will he be leaving? Any time soon?" I spoke quietly as Simon's room was dark and it was almost midnight.

"Simon's doing great, Tabitha. He's probably going to be transferred to Step-down tomorrow," Kai replied.

At that moment Simon stirred, and called for Kai. He then disappeared into the darkened room but was back a few seconds later. "Simon wants to see you," Kai said. "He heard you talking to me in the doorway and wants to see what you look like! Sure hope he doesn't get scared and have a relapse!"

"Hilarious Kai! Ha! Ha!" I said as I stepped into Simon's room. Simon looked at me.

"I knew that was you outside. Your voice. I wanted to see what you look like!" he mumbled.

I smiled. My English accent never allowed me to get away with much! "That's amazing Simon. All the time I looked after you, you were heavily sedated," I said. I leaned against the wall and chatted with him about what had gone on during those first two nights when he was really critical and then finished up with, "Okay, Simon. It's getting late. Must be going."

Simon stopped me. "Thank you for stopping by and checking on me," he said. "And for looking after me too," he added.

I felt good inside. "It was my pleasure, Simon. I'm glad you'll be home soon. That's great news," and I left his room.

* * *

Over the past 20 years I had learned to say little phrases like "It's my pleasure," and "You are welcome," instead of a plain, "Okay," or "Thanks" as so often the stiff-upper-lip-Brit might. Learning to show people that I valued their appreciation was an interesting journey for me, and still is. Coming to live in the US when English is your mother tongue, can be challenging. A strange happening repeatedly occurred when I was in a store, or office, or bank. The clerk would suddenly say, "Oh…I love your accent. Say something more."

At first I was taken aback by such a comment, but as they kept coming, I became annoyed by what I thought were flattering, syrupy remarks. I created a few smart, mental rebuffs, but later decided to take my bad attitude in hand, and developed appropriate, moderately long responses, that in giving them, I would grant the person their wish. I would smile and say, "I have been blessed with an English accent. Thank you for asking me to say something more," or, "I am not so sure my children would agree with you, but they aren't here now!" Sometimes I would ask them, "Would you like a spoonful of sugar in your tea, Ma'am?" or "Did you know that the rain in Spain stays mainly in the plain?" Satisfied with my answer, life went on. Now I am prepared, even though I still feel the request is somewhat weird.

* * *

"Well, I'll be darned, Kai," I said as I emerged from the room. "Simon is proof positive that chemically sedated kids can recognize voices, and remember them. Probably he understood some of what I said too!"

"I thought you'd find that interesting. Not that anyone misses your face, Tabitha!"

"Oh really?"

Kai laughed.

"Well, Simon just confirmed that we should always be careful as to what we say within earshot of a sedated kid, no matter the accent!"

* * *

How we transport a kid to the PICU is determined by the Pediatric Intensivist on service at the time the call comes in. He, or she, takes into consideration many factors when deciding, including the reported condition of the kid, the availability of ground and air transportation, and the distance to cover. When flying for a patient is the best choice, the pilot actually has the final say as to whether it is safe for the Team to take off, or not.

Like many other experienced PICU nurses, I rotated on and off the Transport Team schedule and well know the adrenalin rush of a transport call, and of bringing a young kid to the PICU for medical care that is unavailable at smaller, referring hospitals.

* * *

It was 2.30 AM and I was asleep —but on call. I woke to the jingle of my phone on the nightstand. "You're flying to South Coast, Tabitha. The kid is nine months old. Respiratory distress. It looks bad. Get in here, girl." Despite having gotten only three hours sleep since the previous transport, I had to be on the floor within 30-minutes. It was required. And I was.

Picking up the Transport Communication Sheet I read that the kid, Sabrina, was not doing well. There was no way a small hospital could care for a little kid in severe respiratory distress. The Team would probably intubate her and get her back to the PedsICU ASAP. Within five minutes of arriving on the floor, the Team was ready to leave for the helipad. Hauling our heavy bag of equipment on wheels behind me, I jogged along beside the other team members, a Pediatrician and an RT, towards the peds helipad. The bag was stuffed with IV fluids and drugs, tubings, interosseous access needles, intubation equipment and more. We replenished supplies after each call and locked the bag in the Transport Room, ready for the next trip.

Forty-five minutes after take-off we landed at the referring hospital. A patient transport courier rushed out of the ER pushing an empty gurney onto the helipad. We heaved our bags onto it and headed for the Emergency Room. Rushing into the cubicle the nurse directed us to, we found Sabrina sitting on her mother's lap smiling.

"Sabrina?" I asked the mother.

The mother nodded her head. The child was Sabrina. The Team looked at each other blankly.

"Is this Sabrina?" asked the RT again, sure that there must be a mistake. It was Sabrina. The "critically ill" kid we were going to transport to PedsICU ASAP was smiling up at us, enjoying the attention. I felt the adrenalin drain from me as I carefully assessed our happy little patient. Sabrina was the right kid, but transporting her by air? What could be the reason? There was little of real significance to note about her except that she had supplemental oxygen running at two whole liters a minute! What a fiasco! And yet, what if it had been a different story?

AJ had been a different story. A very different story and a transport was etched into my mind.

* * *

It had been a busy Transport Schedule and I would be off-duty at 7 AM. I had rolled into bed around 3 AM confident that I would sleep until my alarm went off in the morning so that I could get my daughter off to school. Two Transport Teams team-tagged, so it was highly unlikely that I would have to go out again. *Oh the joy!* The other team had to have gone out before I would be called again. But I was totally wrong.

My phone rang. It was 5.15 AM.

"You're on, Tabitha. Sorry. It's only Rialto Community. You'll be back home in time to get up!"

That was no consolation.

We arrived at Rialto Community in less than 20 minutes, just as the sun rose for another day of solid heat. We rapidly rolled through the ER, which was unusually busy for that time of day. Getting to AJ's cubicle, we found the source of the business. He was bucking the ventilator as staff hung on to four-point restraints. Probably a restraint had got lose and had been recaptured only minutes earlier. A family of too many were talking excitedly and standing to the side, and in the way, as a sedative, probably, was being pushed to quieten him down a little.

His nurse was distressed.

"He's been like this for the last half hour…so glad you got here."

I learned that AJ was eleven years old and a healthy kid until a day ago. Three days ago the family took a trip to the hot springs and he had had a blast. Yesterday he had become confused and agitated and in the early evening he was acting so bizarrely that his parents brought him in — just in time. At first the fever had been controlled with Tylenol® but then it would soar off the charts. A bucket of half-melted ice with wash-cloths dangling over the side stood forlornly on the counter nearby. A few wash cloths lay on the bed, now warm, next to him.

The ER nurse explained that when AJ became somnolent, his breathing rate dropped dangerously low, and consequently his oxygen levels went down into the 80s, enough for them to decide to intubate him and send him to Inland Valley —quickly. His neurological status was obviously the most concerning and Rialto wouldn't be able to look after him. The labs showed he had an infection of some sort –hence the raging fever.

We had the papers signed by his parents, who were going to follow us, and him on board for the short trip to IVCH in record time. The 12-minute race to the medical center felt like time stood still as the RT and I attempted to keep him intubated and secured to the gurney. Luckily the roads weren't clogged with traffic. The time couldn't go fast enough. Documentation would have to wait. I had no hands to write with. The monitor would contain all the information I would need. I would print out the q 5-minute vital signs and then build my documentation around them *after* the fact.

We rushed the gurney into Room 8 where a team of tired night nurses, two RTs and a Resident were waiting for us. Seeing AJ, a wild, skinny kid in restraints and as strong as a raging ox, fired them up and he was wrestled into the scales and then onto the bed, and carefully restrained.

A brief report to the night nurses was followed by a full report to a day nurse who had arrived a little early and was ready to get her day going. The disheveled Attending, who had already had a bad night, got to the station in record minutes and I knew that I was leaving AJ in good hands. I was relieved.

Documenting the transport, re-filling the transport bag and locking it up for the last time meant that I wasn't home until my daughter was at school. *Oh well…*

I returned to the unit after a long nap, late in the afternoon. I still had some catch-up to do.

Sauntering down to Station Two I looked into Room 8. It was sparkling clean, and empty.

Faye, the day nurse to whom I had given report saw me.

"He didn't make it," she said. "AJ died a few hours ago."

I was gobsmacked. I had only brought AJ in nine hours earlier. How could this have happened? What about his parents? Didn't he have a little sister too? How were they?

Two days later, I learned that AJ had developed amebic encephalitis after snorting water up his nose while playing in the hot springs. The ameba had travelled into his brain and AJ was gone.

As I drove home, thankful to be able to sleep this night, I wondered what could have been done differently. How would his sister see life after enjoying such an innocent time at the hot-springs? Who had first suggested going to the hot-springs for fun? Were they to blame for AJ dying? Where was God when they were enjoying a family outing?

Sometimes there are no answers, at least no answers that bring relief. Only pain and emptiness.

* * *

We loaded Sabrina into the helicopter to receive a "higher level of care" at Inland Valley, and set off for home. The Team was quiet all the way back to the Children's Hospital, thankful that Sabrina was not as critical as had been thought, –and not a bit like AJ. We had little to do on the flight, except to lose sleep! Sabrina was a cute, healthy little kid, and oblivious to the excitement of her first helicopter ride.

Who paid the humongous bill to transport her was another matter, but we admitted her to the Step-down ICU for observation. The Transport Team should not have been called for Sabrina, especially to go by air, but we followed the Intensivists orders based on the information he had received from the referring hospital. *Oh well, that was a serendipitous transport call –but not worth the loss of sleep.*

* * *

Many of the PICU kids are prayed-for kids. The wall-hanging at the end of the long, central corridor says, "Life is Precious, Handle it With Prayer." It is a constant reminder as to how fragile many of our kids are. They are prayed for by their nurses, physicians and other members of the health care team, and by their parents and family members too, and most of them recover. Some kids survive the most horrific happenings, or are saved from abusive situations and in so doing, find new strength and joy in their lives. Being in PICU might even change their life permanently, turning an unexpected storm in their life, into a golden opportunity.

Stephanie, a little 10-month-old kid, was adopted by one of the PICU staff after being abused by her mother's boyfriend. She would always have deficits as a result of her injuries, but now she has the opportunities any little child should have, and a bright future ahead of her. Dr. Caleb King is now a well-loved pediatric oncologist. He lost a leg to cancer when he was a kid, and is now treating cancer kids himself. Surviving cancer turned his life in a completely new direction.

And some kids change their parent's lives.

Carolyn's 14-year-old daughter died of cancer. That changed Carolyn's life forever. It was devastating but Carolyn is now an oncology nurse. "I would have never become a nurse if Sarah hadn't died of cancer," she said. "The cancer roller-coaster was terrible, but I found amazing nurses on the hemoc floor, and in PedsICU."

Carolyn entered nursing school a year after Sarah died, and since graduating, true to her word, she has worked on the pediatric hemoc unit. "This is my calling," Carolyn said. "I will never work anywhere else. Every day I work as a nurse I honor my daughter."

* * *

Like most nurses, PICU nurses are adaptable –they have to be. Our kids can be new-born, weighing in at a mere three kilos, or they can be giants like Jaden, and an adult size. Some patients are admitted with a simple diagnosis like a ruptured appendix, while others, like AJ, challenge us with extremely rare diagnoses, or really bizarre circumstances surround their admission.

* * *

Problems arise when a pediatric patient is a geriatric, in our view. We expect our patients to range in age from birth to 17 years, so there had to be a very good explanation as to why a 20-year-old was to be admitted to a PICU bed! Pediatric nurses do not like looking after adults. Even kids over 16 years of age are somewhat rare in PICU, as they can be admitted to an adult ICU. In placing them on an adult floor, a pediatric bed is freed-up for a real kid. Age is, therefore, an important factor in our pediatric population, but some PedsICU nurses also apply the tongue-in-cheek standard, the Hair Rule.

"If there's hair anywhere other than on the head, they're not our kids!"

The Hair Rule might be over-ridden when a fourteen-year-old, who is already a parent (and therefore legally an adult), needs to be admitted. But these situations are rare.

An uproar broke out in the Nurses Lounge when the Charge Nurse announced that one of our patients was 23 years old. "Twenty-three years old!" "No way!" "She's not a pediatric patient. She's a geriatric patient!" "I'm not taking her," were the responses to this shocking announcement.

The Charge broke in. "Okay...Okay. I hear you guys, but she had emergency surgery, and we had to take her because there were no adult beds in the Medical Center...zero beds, nada, zilch. We had no choice." With us now listening, she continued. "It will be for only one night. She'll be transferred out tomorrow."

Mil eventually took Sandra, the 23-year-old, and what a great list she had! However, there was another slight problem. Sandra had a four-month-old, breast-feed baby in tow! Usually the problem on the PedsICU is that of sibling visitation, not an infant visiting his mother. Should we let Sandra's mom, the baby's grandmother, bring Sandra's little son in to breastfeed for each feed? Sandra could not go off the floor to nurse him in the Visitor's Lounge, but we didn't want a healthy little baby picking up an infection that was lurking on our floor. In the end, there was only one reasonable answer: Little Harry would stay the night in his mom's room, and be a "boarder."

The shift went well and Mil enjoyed keeping an eye on a cute, happy, smiling, healthy little four-month-old and his mother, and the next day Sandra reluctantly left the unit after a bed opened-up for her on an adult floor.

"I never thought it could be so fun being a kid again!" she said as she was wheeled down the hallway.

And then there was Darryl.

* * *

Darryl just made it onto our floor. He was 17 years old, which made him a pediatric patient. He had advanced muscular dystrophy. Many MD kids don't survive to seventeen despite frequent admissions and improved medical support for them at home. Their future can still be bleak.

Over the years, PedsICU nurses get to know a few MD kids and their families, and develop lasting relationships. Many of them have Primary Nurses who care for them on every admission. However Darryl was not a frequent flier. He was an unknown but, because of increasing respiratory weakness, he was admitted.

Darryl lived his life in an iron lung. The energy he used breathing, resulted in him having a big personality within an emaciated body, and time was running out for him. Darryl, like all our advanced MD kids, wanted his limbs placed in precisely the right position for his comfort. The day he was admitted, he was exceedingly distressed. "I am getting married in three days," he said weakly to the Resident, Mark. "I've got to be out of here by then."

"I don't think so Darryl," Mark said quietly. "You will need to be here longer than two days. We will need to work you up —and that takes time." Intellectually, Darryl knew that the doctor was right, but his time, his life was limited.

"I must get home. The wedding's three days away. Everything is planned."

Darryl eventually gave in. He was too ill to fight anyone. He needed to be admitted for urgent treatment, and when Kaitlyn, his fiancé heard the news that the wedding had been delayed, she cried. Stroking Darryl's head which protruded from the iron lung, Kaitlyn then pulled herself together and said, "Don't worry, Honey. We'll get married next week, when you are home."

Shelli, his day-shift nurse, heard this sad reality, and decided to do something about it. She marched down to the Nurse Manager's office to plead Darryl and Kaitlyn's case.

"Darryl's not going to live long, and we don't have any protocols forbidding our patients from getting married so...let's do it!" she announced. "Let's do the wedding here!"

Shelli won her case. Her enthusiasm was contagious, and three days later a team of nurses decorated Darryl's room and brought in extra chairs for guests. Darryl grinned when his beautiful bride walked into his room to Mendelssohn's Wedding March, and the ceremony began. One of our Hospital Chaplains performed the ceremony, and a small reception followed in the space where carts and equipment usually stood.

The wedding was a first —and would probably be the only one to take place in the PedsICU. But it was a beautiful, joyful, occasion, and worth the hassle. After the celebrations, the housekeepers cleaned up the confetti and rice, and Darryl's medication regimens and treatments returned to normal. A few days later, Darryl was discharged home, a married man, to his wife.

Less than a year after Darryl's wedding, a PICU nurse saw a small obituary in the local paper stating that Darryl had died peacefully. She brought it in and pinned it on the board in the Nurses Lounge. "I'm glad we went ahead with the wedding," Shelli said as she read the obit, and wiped a tear from her eye. "I will never forget that wedding. It was all good. We gave Darryl a few extra days being the person he wanted to be –married."

Shelli was right.

* * *

Our frequent fliers often leave a mark on us too, at least Carl did. "Back again Carl?" the secretary asked Carl as he slid by in his wheelchair with his mom trailing behind him. "You sure have grown since we last saw you. You're in 14 this time."

Carl's mom, Fiona, slowed down to talk to the Charge Nurse and find out if Carl's Primary Nurse was working. By this time, Carl was way down the hall and turning right into Station Three. He knew the geography of the floor, and the ropes. "Carl will be 17 in two weeks," his mom continued. "This might be his last time here."

"I hope not," the Unit Secretary said with a smile. "Not that we want him ill of course, but we sure miss our kids when they grow up and leave us. If he's ever on the adult floors, you *must* drop by and let us know how things are going. I am sure Luanne would want to visit with you."

The unavoidable advance into maturity automatically changes the connections we have made with our frequent-flier kids and their parents. At eighteen, our kids are tossed into the hazardous waters of adult medical care, unsteadily making their journey through unchartered waters with new medical teams. When they move on, it leaves a hole in our hearts. The relationship may survive in an altered form, but eventually it is lost.

"Luanne isn't on today, Fiona," Corrine, the Charge Nurse said to Carl's mom. "But she'll be here tomorrow, and for the next three days. Carl will get to have her then."

"That's good," Fiona said. "He's looking forward to updating her about school, and a new girlfriend," she said with a wink. "This time it's only a tune-up, so he shouldn't be in for more than a few days." Parents of these frequent fliers know everything about their child, so the Team is well advised to listen to them.

"Well, I'm glad to hear that. It's been about 18-months since we saw Carl, isn't it?" Corrine had an uncanny way of remembering our frequent-flier admissions fairly accurately.

"You're right. He was last here 20-months ago. It was a nasty pneumonia. Do you remember? He goes to the Vent Clinic every month, and sometimes more often, but this time he's getting a major tune-up."

Many more of our admissions are frequent-fliers, kids who, because they have a chronic medical condition, occasionally require sophisticated monitoring, or a change in therapy as they out-grow treatment modalities. Then, if they have a Primary Nurse, she will be looking out for them. She wants to get re-connected because they often develop long-term friendships.

* * *

The majority of our kids, however, are regular, fun-loving kids who are getting on with life, totally unaware of the dangers surrounding them. Suddenly, life takes a nasty turn and throws their parents, and loved ones, into a tortuous vortex of distress, anxiety, and recrimination. Even though they were doing their best as parents, something went tragically wrong on their watch.

"I don't think this place should be here," a young father said to me as he stood at the front of the unit. "It's all wrong." He was upset. *Well, if we weren't here, your son might be dead,* I thought.

"Unfortunately…" I started to say. "Unfortunately…"

"What I mean is kids shouldn't need to be in an ICU."

I understood his point, but it was irrelevant. PedsICUs are, *unfortunately*, very necessary and save thousands of kids' lives every year. His son's life —and many more kids' lives, become little miracles after coming to us under some very dark circumstances. It's what PedsICUs are about: Saving kids' lives now, so that they can have a future.

PICU Kids, Our Heroes

CHAPTER 2

The Set-Up

I WAS ALMOST LATE –AGAIN! I lived life on the edge of time, and being late was never on my agenda. On time? Yes. Early? No. *Don't waste my time, it is in short supply*. Time management had been drummed into me as a child, although the term "time management" had not be coined then. *Be on time, Tabitha. Be reliable. Don't waste time, Tabitha, because Satan finds work for idle hands to do!* Now, as an adult, Satan would not get a look-in with respect to me wasting time. However, time-wasting wasn't the only "sin" in my repertoire.

Swishing up to the parking lot, I slid almost onto the bumper of the car in front. If I stuck to his tail, I wouldn't have to take all of the 10-seconds to plunge my badge into the card reader, get in gear and drive in. It would be done for me. Perfect. Like adhesive to dentures, I hung on and snuck in under the barricade before it dropped down. *Whew! Perfect timing –again.* I swerved around the tight corners and slid into my slot, one that I had used so many times that I could have hung my shingle over the spot – except that security would not have been happy! Grabbing my backpack from the back seat, I slammed the door shut and set off at a brisk pace for PedsICU.

Rushing up the five flights of stairs, *why go by the elevator when you have legs, Tabitha?* –and having not been out for a run today, the stairs were my exercise. A quick turn by the elevators –and I slammed my card into the card reader. I was on time –just. *Perfecto!*

An adult male was hurling four-letter words generously at the intercom as he threw a few sharp kicks and punches on the door. *Welcome to another shift!* Why do nurses call in early to find out what is going on? Being on time was more than soon enough for me. Isn't 12-hours of stress enough?

The Set Up

I heard Connie's voice crackling through the intercom. "It's change of shift…" Twice a day, all family members were asked to leave the unit for an hour to give the nurses time to give, or get report, and check out our kids. Heaving my bulging back-pack up onto my shoulder I pushed against the door, consciously keeping visitors from sliding in behind me, and marched towards the front desk.

"If anyone else calls me and asks me what is the best assignment tonight, or if so-and-so kid is still here, I think I will scream," Connie said as she stored a big bag of who-knows-what under her desk. Nona, the off-going secretary, waited for her to get upright.

"That's because you are so nice," chided Jill, a night-shift nurse who was passing in front of Connie's desk ahead of me on her way to the Nurses Lounge. "Everyone loves you!" she added. Connie smiled at the whopping lie, and scooted her chair up to the desk. "No, Jill. I'm their *Contact*," she said emphatically signing quotes in the air, "and I know NOTHING," she yelled jokingly.

The phone rang and Connie grabbed it. "No, Room 14 is no longer here, and Room 12 has been paired with a new patient and —I'm not answering another call!" she said as she slammed the phone down. "What's her point?" Connie said turning to Nona who was still waiting to give report. "Beth's always late. Why doesn't she turn up on time? Then she'd get a choice!" Connie turned her back to the phone, and began to pay full attention to Nona who was anxious to go home.

Another night shift was underway. Connie had given early callers the low-down on what could be the best assignment —and who they should avoid. Connie had no *real* inside knowledge, but some nurses thought that calling in early to get her prognostications, was worth it. They might get the edge on another nurse and corner the best list merely because they believed Connie did have foresight, and called early. But I knew it was empty air –usually. My interrogation for Connie was two words, "Which room?"

"Twelve," Connie said. She knew what my question meant.

"Thanks." *Sure don't want Room 12!*

As was common, frenetic activity flashed across Station One as I hung a right to the Nurses Lounge. The busyness on Station One might not be an accurate predictor of the next 12-hour shift. It probably reflected the usual nose-dive many shifts take in the last hour, although some nurses refused to work on Station One whether they saw extreme activity or not. It was common for a frazzled secretary to be answering the phone and talking to relatives outside the unit door, while tracking a nurse over the intercom, and entering STAT orders into the computer. But busy or not, it is too late to call in sick when you are there, and I wasn't one of those nurses who categorically refused to work on Station One saying, "I'll not work there unless someone puts a gun to my head. Phones, visitors, doorbells and patients. Never. I'm not working there!"

Another possible tell-tale predictor of a hectic start to a shift is meeting the Transport Team hauling their bags towards the exit, on their way to pick up a critical kid. If that isn't bad enough, you might spot the Transport Nurse from the previous transport call catching up on paperwork before going home. That means that somewhere on the floor it is busy, and somewhere else on the floor it is going to be super busy when the Transport Team returns.

What was tonight going to be like? More nurses than usual had leaned over the secretary's desk to check the status of the unit –but I'd know soon enough.

On the good side, the Code Blue alarm wasn't ringing relentlessly, and there was no Stat Cart flying through Station One with a crop of medical personnel in quick pursuit. Nor was the staff from the Organ Procurement Agency huddled over cell phones in the room adjacent to the Nurses Lounge reminding us of the uncomfortable fact that some of our kids die. On the other hand, their presence would tell us that we have some wonderful, self-sacrificing parents who donate their kid's organs to save other children's lives.

However tonight, in a flash, I caught sight of intense activity around Room 3. *Hmmm...new critical kid on Station One after all. So that's where it's happening tonight –to begin with.*

I didn't want Room 12 for sure, and really critical kids were still in Rooms 16 and 17. Presumably, they were still circling the proverbial drain. They had been doing this for two whole weeks. Every shift had been a small miracle, and tonight they were still alive. But it wouldn't last forever. Maybe tonight would be the last night –at least for one of them. We all knew it would eventually happen. They would be sucked down into a dark, deep void where no family wants to go, and where emptiness, pain, and deep wounds attack bereaved parents. The only real question was as to who would go first. I knew that. The doctors knew that. The secretary knew that. Everyone knew that —except for their families, who still clung to hope and the chance of a miracle for their child.

I dashed into the Nurses Lounge and dropped my back-pack on the floor. *On time.* Nurses' bags bulged with magazines and books that wouldn't be read, and school work that would not be completed. The atmosphere was serious. There wasn't the usual chatter, and the television was off, making the room unusually quiet —even ominous. All the nurses seemed to have a sure knowledge that the next 12-hours would not be a bundle of fun. They were waiting for the Charge Nurse to come in to "assign" lists – late. Having to wait a long time for the assignments was another bad sign.

We knew all about shifts that turn into shifts from hell. Some creep up on us almost imperceptibly until we feel overwhelmed by the extreme pressure of the crazy situation. Other hell-holes explode in a single moment, with no intimation of what is about to happen. Too late, the shit hits the fan, propelling us with our kids, towards invisible disaster, or not.

It's shifts that start with uncertainty and a lousy aura, that make us question why we choose to work in such a high-stress environment, 12-hours at a time, for months and years on end. The answer is defined in as many ways as there are PedsICU nurses, multiplied by the number of shifts we work.

"I love being a nurse, and I love kids." *Simple*

"Kids don't deserve to be in an ICU, so I want to help them get home again." *Agreed —so let someone else do it.*

"I can't stand adults. They usually get what they ask for." *Hmmm…*

"I don't know why –but I'm never leaving." *Sure…but just you wait another 6-months. You won't be so naïve then.*

"I love kids, and we have the best team of nurses." *Yeah, that's true.*

"There's never a dull moment." *Exactly.*

"I need the money." *So? Don't nurses working elsewhere get paid?*

"It's fun – except on the bad days, but everybody has bad days at work." *True, but do we have to have so many bad days?*

We rationalize our concerns because shifts are only 12-hours long, after which we go home and forget about work –except sometimes we can't forget about it. It's impossible. Being stressed and anxious at work, and even before work, is acceptable to a certain degree, but there are times when the severity of apprehension overtakes some of us, and causes horrible emotional upset and physiological symptoms. We should be concerned about this, and we are.

We've seen burn-out happen before, but so far we've been okay. We've been able to deal with the stress but we keep an eye on our colleagues for evidence of burnout and stress-fatigue, and ignore ourselves until it hits us. Too late!

So, we sit waiting to learn our fate for the next 12-hours. Wondering. Talking.

Last night Station Four looked terrible, really terrible. Marci was still hanging on in Room 17. She had been a healthy 15-year-old kid until three weeks before. We admitted her with breathing difficulties and an enlarged abdomen. She was a good kid according to her family —a polite, popular, pretty, high-school sophomore. Now she was so critically ill that she was on a 2-to-1 list, with two nurses assigned to her care each shift. For 10-days it had been like that, as Marci continued to sink deeper into the gaping abyss. No one was sure how deep the abyss was, but most thought that the bottom had been reached a long time ago, only to learn that they were wrong. There were still greater depths into which she could plunge. The conventional ventilator had been replaced by a high-frequency vent, which chugged monotonously, shaking her lungs in an endeavor to bring about her recovery. It was a bad sign, and her pretty face was like that of many seriously ill kids, bloated. Her formerly healthy, athletic legs were like sticks, and multiple med-fusion pumps lined the bedtable and IVs hung from poles, their tubings crisscrossing her deathly-ill body. And yet, no one knew *exactly* what her problem was.

But Marci was still here and we had avoided many near disasters. Perhaps she really would turn the corner – perhaps tonight.

The Team had worked Marci up for many obscure — and common diagnoses, only to find none of them an exact fit. Perhaps it was lupus, or maybe an infection caught from contaminated water when she visited her extended family in Uruguay, perhaps a new strain of the Ebola virus. As problems surfaced destabilizing her fragile condition, the docs initiated new treatments. Keeping her alive another day was the goal, but hope vaporized as the days passed and there was no sign of a miraculous recovery. Her being alive today was a miracle in itself, and just enough to keep a flicker of hope glimmering in her family's heart.

Next to Marci, in Room 16, was Ricardo, a 7-year-old with leukemia. Multiple relapses dogged him, and he too was on a high-frequency vent. He was fighting for his life. Both Ricardo and Marci had been circling the drain, but neither had been sucked down –yet. Tonight though, the staff was sure one would go –but everyone had been convinced of that three shifts ago, two shifts ago -and even 12-hours ago, and they were both still here, struggling to stay alive.

The real money was on Marci, as her parents had recently made her a complete No Code. There would be no thumping on her chest, no electric shocks and no medications to bring her back. She would be allowed to die peacefully, if one could call being hooked up to so much equipment, peaceful. There was nothing more medically that would be done to sustain her life as medications supporting her blood pressure were already maxed-out, and she was on 100% oxygen on the high-frequency vent. Marci's parents had made the most difficult decision that any parent could be asked to make. And yet her family continued to pray for a miracle.

When I last saw Marci's parents so distraught and sad, I thought of my daughter who was two years older than Marci. What if my daughter were Marci? How would I survive such an ordeal? Could I have made my daughter a DNR? By God's grace I would never have to make that decision, and yet the possibility was real. Occasionally, nurses imagine being forced to make such a decision, but us knowing something intellectually isn't the same as having to make the actual choice —a life and death choice for your child. A sad fact too, is that every parent's decision to make their child a No Code is criticized by a well-meaning relative or friend, who has never walked in their moccasins. These relative are incredibly ill-equipped to voice their opinions when they have not experienced the asphyxiating fear that comes to parents as the noose tightens around their necks, and their child drifts towards certain death.

In reality, the only unknown left in Marci and Ricardo's unhappy situations was "when," not "if." Ricardo was more likely to hang on for a few more days, but only time would tell.

So much for Station Four. No wonder Ellen was taking so long to divvy up the lists.

Station Five wasn't a happy place to work either. Nadine was 17 years old. It was unusual for us to have two such elderly pediatric kids on the unit at one time and she too looked deathly ill, and after two surgeries, she was making minimal progress. Her obscure medical history and unusual symptoms baffled the Team, but the distinct suspicion of her having a highly contagious disease meant that she was forced to remain under Contact Precaution Isolation. Her family, and all her care givers had to gown, mask and glove whenever they entered her room. Caring for her was a very exacting job, and nothing seemed to add up. Nadine's parents faced an additional worry. Nadine had a young son at home.

Stations Two and Three were both busy, but all the patients were holding their own at present —which left Station One, with the mystery patient in Room 3 whom I saw was already very busy. No wonder the Nurses Lounge was quiet as nurses waited apprehensively to learn their sentence for the next 12-hours.

As luck would have it, I got David, in Room 1, again. I'd had David the night before. He was also on a high-frequency vent, but his prognosis was good. He was sure to make it home eventually. It was agreed that I would help out with the new kid in Room 3, if need be. I read the brief report written on the Master Report Sheet and then took the card bearing David's name. He was stable. All should be well. Anyhow, it was too late to hand back my assignment, and besides, all the other assignments looked much worse. I had lucked out. I got report from the day-shift nurse at the bedside and then she left. It was brief, but that was okay because I knew David.

"Hi David, I'm back again," I said. "Glad your mom was in for a while today... That must have been nice for you."

David was intubated, sedated and paralyzed, but I kept up the chatter as I performed my shift assessment, checked his lines, the ventilator and monitors, and tidied his room. "Stan's your RT tonight, David," I went on. "He's a good storyteller... I'll ask him to tell you the story about how his daughter found a rattlesnake in their backyard, and what happened. It's a great story. Want to hear it?"

David was five-years-old and a sickler who was an infrequent, frequent-flier. All he needed at this stage of his admission was time. Time to heal. After that, he would go home, cured for a while —but likely to return eventually. *Thank you, God, for one stable kid.*

CHAPTER 3

Room 3

I HAD A GOOD DEAL. My kid was stable. I knew David, a little sickler, and it could be a no-sweat night for me. Whatever else might happen on the floor was anyone's guess –but I would help out in Room 3 if I had to.

I glanced into Room 3 and counted six nurses, two doctors and two respiratory therapists in the room —a crowd for sure. Two extra nurses, adult ICU Resource Nurses, were loitering outside the room ready to run to the pharmacy for infusions, draw up medications, or do whatever needed to be done to stabilize the new kid.

Probably the Supe had stationed them there to help us out. *Very thoughtful of her, especially at the beginning of the shift.* As to what was going on in Room 3 was a puzzle with too many missing pieces, but for sure, the little girl was another critically ill kid. I learned that the team had transported her to IVCH by air and that her parents had not arrived yet. *Not a good situation.* Her admission papers were obviously incomplete and we had to use a substitute medical record number, *another problem*, especially as specimens had to be labeled by hand. This could be an exacting job when multiple requisitions had to be completed.

The door slid open. Most likely a central line had been placed as I saw a bag of blood samples being brought out of the room. One of the Resource Nurses took the bag. A radiology tech rumbled in with his machine, the room emptied briefly and then the x-ray machine growled back to its parking spot, half-way down the hall. Hopefully the central line was in the correct position so that labs would be easy to draw and meds, infusions (and the transfusion of blood products), could be given quickly. The admission was progressing well.

I quickly learned that Briella was the new kid in Room 3. She was six years old and was on a conventional ventilator, so probably her lungs weren't her major problem

—at least not at the moment. She was well sedated and calm. Blood, however, was a high priority. Bags of blood were brought in, checked and pushed through the central line. This was followed by plasma, albumen, and other fluids. *What could be her diagnosis?*

As interested as I was in Briella, David was my only patient. I suctioned him, rechecked his IVs and monitors and tipped up the urometer. Forty-six milliliters of clear, yellow urine. *Good.* Washing my hands, I looked past Room 2 and into the front corner of Room 3. Still busy.

Suddenly a fine, rapid, high-pitched beeping sound reverberated around the floor. The Code Blue alarm. Where was the Code? Room 16 ... Room 17... Nadine's room? With the sound drilling in my ears, I realized that not one of those answers was correct. The intercom broke into my room. "Code Blue, Room 3. Code Blue, Room 3."

The din of the alarm did not last long. It had not been a matter of pushing the Code button and hoping the team would arrive promptly, because everyone who was required to attend a Code was already there. The adult ICU nurses were now focused. They would be needed.

With the Code being so near the start of a shift, there were no free nurses to rush from their station to help.

Anyhow, nurses had to be on each station for safety, and all the stations were busy. I still had work to do for David, but, as no PICU nurses materialized, I realized I had been signed up to help in Room 3. I re-thought my workload. Documentation could wait until later. Everything was in order in David's room. His blood pressure was stable. He was chemically paralyzed and sedated and was therefore comfortable, and I knew his alarms were set. I'd have to go.

I beckoned one of the adult Resource Nurses over and asked her to watch David. She was quick to agree. I knew her to be an excellent ICU nurse, but her specialty was adult cardiothoracic surgery, and she had never worked in the PICU before. Our floor was also geographically different from the adult floors, so this would be an added challenge for her.

"David's stable, and has no meds due for over an hour. He's sedated and paralyzed. He has an antibiotic running. It's almost through. Just turn it off when it's done, please." I gave her a quick run-down. She agreed to sit in David's room and watch the monitors. She would call for help if something happened.

Relieved of my job, I wound my way into the crowded room and volunteered to take over documenting the Code. I liked documenting. The Code Sheet required me to list medications, check boxes as they were given, document vital signs (or the lack of them) and when chest compressions started and stopped, bagging et cetera. The Code clock, situated on a column above Briella's head, kept track of the Code's duration —and no one had begun to document the Code. Chest compressions had been started by the PICU staff and another nurse was drawing up meds and an RT was bagging. I took my place to the left of the bed, near the activity. I had to see everything as it happened —plus see the monitor on the Code Cart. Being very near-sighted, I wore strong glasses and standing on the periphery of the activity wasn't an option for me.

2012...Compressions?...Check. Bagging?...Check.

"What's her weight?" "Has epi been given, guys?"

I worked my way across the sheet and down the columns. Briella had no blood pressure to record. *So much for vital signs.*

Nurses and ancillary staff ran in and out of the room as the Intensivist snapped out orders, keeping the Code Team hopping, intent on doing everything without delay. Ten minutes into the Code, the familiar *ding-dong* of the intercom rang out into Room 3. A hush came over the team as the Charge Nurse who was with us connected directly with Room 17, Marie's room.

"Marie's expired," Marie's nurse relayed simply. The team breathed again, not missing a beat, so as to keep the Code running smoothly. God must be looking out for us, I thought. It was a blessing that Marie had been made a "No Code" recently. It meant that nothing had to be done emergently for her, and everyone could concentrate on getting Briella back –soon.

The Charge Nurse cut the connection between the rooms and quietly slipped out, hurrying catty-corner across the floor to Room 17. The inevitable had finally happened, and we had the answer to our questions, "Who?" and "When?"

"Marie. Today –now."

* * *

Marie's death propelled her family into the next stage of their difficult journey. Ellen found the heart-broken family weeping beside their daughter's bed, their arms wrapped around each other as they said the first of many farewells. Tears streamed down her mother's face and the familiar sound of the deepest, most profound inner sobbing that anyone could experience, escaped from yet another heart-broken mother. From this lowest of low positions, the family had to draw an ounce of strength to start them on their long journey from Marie's last breath, to recovery without her —a seemingly impossible task.

Much later, Marie's family left her stiffening, sallow body on the bed and walked one last time down the all-too-familiar hallways, in a daze. I caught sight of them as they turned to leave the floor, exhausted by weeks of fear and uncertainty. Their tear-stained faces told a story of painful loss. They could not see a silver-lined cloud beyond the horizon, because their worst fears had been realized. In a split second their world had changed forever for the worse.

After the family left, Marie was ID'd and bagged in an ugly, off-white, soft plastic shroud. She was zippered in and taken by couriers to the morgue in the covered wagon.

* * *

But for everyone in Room 3, another life hung in the balance, Briella's. She was our newest kid, and we still hadn't got her back.

2022. Chest compressions…Check. Bagging on 100%...Check.

Would she become the second casualty of the night before her parents arrived at the PedsICU? No one had missed a single compression. It was a skill PICU nurses learned by experience –unfortunately, and it was early in Briella's Code. We tried to run every Code like clock-work, and today we had to get Briella back.

I glanced outside the door and saw an unfamiliar face. Another nurse had appeared from who knows where. Apparently, the call for assistance had gone out house-wide to all the ICUs. We could rely on our Supe to get the word out for us. The nurse watched the Code briefly and I stared at her.

"I'm here to make sure no one else dies," she mouthed. *Weird,* I thought, *but thank you, Lord.*

"Thanks," I mouthed back, nodding my head. *Was she ever an angel?*

Peds Codes are intense and drawn out. No 10-minute Codes for our kids, as might happen to a 70-year-old COPD-er in an adult ER. It took us a full 45-minutes to get Briella back as we gave multiple rounds of Code Meds, hundreds of effective chest compressions and breaths, and a million prayers. By the end of the code, I had covered 4 ½ Code Sheets with check marks, numbers, and comments.

Thank you, God. The Code Team dispersed as quickly as they had come. There was more to do elsewhere.

With the crisis over, and Briella somewhat stable, I too left to take back David's care. Thirty minutes later the Attending went home. It wasn't yet midnight, but it felt as if it should be the end of a full shift.

Ellen, the Charge Nurse, came back from Room 17 and started clearing up the mess in Room 3. That was no small task after an unexpected Code on a patient who had been on the unit less than an hour. Everything had to be sorted through. Line placement equipment, intubation kits, towels and empty blood bags. Carefully labeled syringes lined the counters and saline flushes lay in clusters on the top of the cart. Catheters and tubes dangled out of open drawers or lay scattered on the floor after missing their target —the trash can, which was overflowing. Color-coded drawers in the cart were partially emptied of their contents. It was the usual post-code muddle.

We left Briella on the backboard which we had placed under her at the start of the Code to support effective chest compressions —just in case. Tonight wasn't a night to tempt providence.

"You never know," is the concern voiced by nurses who remove the backboard early, only to find that Murphy's-Back-board Law is alive and another Code occurs before they can shove the backboard back in place. Leaving it under the patient was a smart, pre-emptive choice.

* * *

Briella's parents arrived during the Code and had been ushered into the Family Room by the Charge Nurse. From time to time she updated them on the Code's progress and brought them cups of coffee that remained untouched on the small table. They waited, not knowing if their child would live or die.

Shortly after the Code, the Charge Nurse took the distraught parents into Briella's room. They were relieved that their daughter was still alive. Briella's mom cried when she saw her daughter looking so fragile and with lines and tubes coming out of her. Briella looked so helpless. Suddenly, her Mom's legs crumpled beneath her and the Charge Nurse leaned forward, catching her just in time, and helped her to a seat beside Briella's bed. Briella's mom stroked her face amid the chaos of the medical equipment, and kept repeating, "Thank you, God. You're alive. I love you Briella. Thank you, God. You're alive. I love you Briella."

Yes, thank God Briella is alive. Briella has a chance of going home one day. Marie would never be going home. Never.

* * *

Marie's nurse, now relieved of her duties in Room 17, joined Briella's bedside nurse for the rest of the shift, making her a two-to-one.

An hour passed before the Code alarm once again shattered the quiet of the night shift. It was Briella again. However, since the previous Code, the Resident had placed an A-line, and Briella now had two nurses on hand who were ready for anything. They sprang into action as Briella's parents made a quick exit to the Family Room with the Charge Nurse. I became Recorder again, and shortly after the Code started, the Attending rushed in from home to take over from the Resident.

It was déjà vu —and it worked again. This time, Briella was back in 20-minutes. "Textbook Code," her nurse said as she cleared away used equipment and restocked the room.

"Great teamwork everyone! Only 2-full-rounds of meds this time."

It was true, it had been a Textbook Code, but the questions on our minds were, "How long will she last?" and "How many times can we get her back?" We didn't know of course, but at this moment we were stoked, and felt optimistic.

I returned to look after David again. *No more Codes, please, Lord.*

* * *

But the night wasn't over. The Transport Team was out, picking up another kid, by ground. They would be returning within the hour. Marie's nurse, who had been helping in Briella's room, now had to take the new admission on Station Four, in Marie's old room. What a night she was having! At least she would sleep well, I thought. But if Briella Codes again, who will help her nurse this time? There were no spare nurses again.

Ellen had been right about the night. It was rough.

Under the radar, while Briella had been coding and Marie had passed away, Yvonne, a nurse on Station Two, had admitted a four-year-old kid, Stevie, from the ER.

Stevie had a depressed skull fracture from being hit on the head with a baseball bat. He had come through the Peds ER, been admitted quickly to PedsICU, and then gone to surgery. The surgery was quick, and before long he was back in his room with his head swathed in bandages. Yvonne started doing the routine post-operative neurological checks.

"I sure didn't want to have my own little drama going on here," Yvonne joked with Ellen when Ellen came by to check on her. "I thought you had enough going on tonight without me complicating things!" she said. "And it kept me out of Room 3," she added triumphantly.

Stevie's parents had a few hours of intense anxiety, but they relaxed after getting to the PICU and asking Yvonne the usual questions of "How's he doing?" "How are his vital signs?" "When will we get to take him home?" to which she had given the usual answers, "He's doing well... his vital signs are stable, including his neuro checks ... You will need to check with the neurosurgeons, but he'll be here for a few days before being transferred off the floor." Their kid would make it, they were sure –almost. For them the night had been an experience they would never forget, a lesson learned. Coming to the PedsICU was a frontier they had never planned to cross, and which they wanted to leave far, far behind, never to revisit. Their taste of the PICU had been more than enough to satisfy any curiosity they might have had about a PICU!

"We are so thankful that Stevie is going to be alright...so thankful," they said to the secretary as they left, bleary-eyed, at around 5 AM –and they meant it.

For Yvonne, Stevie's admission was a small incident with a successful outcome. He was another lucky kid who had only fractured his skull. He would make it. That was the good part of working in the PICU; kids do make it. Yvonne left the floor that morning tired, but thankful for another great outcome.

* * *

Ricardo was still hanging out in Room 16. One more shift had come and gone, and he was still alive. Possibly the miracle would happen today. But for how much longer would he be so critically ill?

On Station Five Nadine still hovered on the brink of losing her battle. Isolated in her room, physicians and nurses came and peered at her through the glass walls and doors, watching monitors and medications from a distance. She didn't know she was a spectacle, nor how close to death she was balanced.

I gave my report on David to the returning day-shift nurse without my usual panache.

"The good news is that David is still alive," I announced, "and he's probably going onto a conventional vent today." I flicked through his chart and scrolled through his medications. "I guess it is a matter of the same-old neuro checks, vital signs and meds," I droned. "I sure am glad you know all about him already. I don't think I would make it if I had to start from the beginning." *Yawn.*

I picked up my backpack and slung it over my shoulder. Passing through the Charge Nurse's Room, I saw Ellen trying to concentrate on relaying the details about every kid on the floor to the day shift Charge Nurse. Wearied by the pace of the night, her voice lacked luster as she described the antics of each Station. It surely has been a night from hell.

All the nurses appeared wasted as they dragged their feet homeward at the end of a very rough shift. They were exhausted, but relieved to be going home to recharge their batteries.

As I trailed out, I passed the mural on the wall showing happy children blowing bubbles, laughing and playing hide and seek. How ironic! There would be no bubble blowing for Marie, but Briella and Stevie still had a chance. PedsICU had given them a new hold on life and hope. When courage is all but gone, the PICU team fans the weakest flicker of hope into a living flame —usually, and the hope of another miracle happening keeps bringing the Team back for the next shift. In essence, PedsICU is often a type of manufacturing plant that generates hope —a hope factory.

CHAPTER 4

Good Luck, Bad Luck

I ENJOY GOOD HEALTH. I am blessed. During my childhood, we often moved to a different house but always lived in small villages, in the countryside. Without having a car, I walked to friends' houses to play, or bicycled if needs be. My mother, a single mother, bought cottages that were somewhat derelict and between 50 and 300-years-old, and, with the help of contractors, we modernized them, created beautiful gardens, and sold them at a profit. We survived, even though moving the household resulted in me attending five different primary (elementary) schools.

Changing schools was difficult, but that was life and I made it. I don't know what my mother would have done if it were today, as there are no cottages to snap up and make a profit on.

At twelve, I started attending the grammar school which was about 10-miles away. It was for girls. The bus stop was two miles from my home, so my sister and I biked there, stashed our bikes with others' bikes at a kind lady's home, and got on the bus to go to school. These were busses for the public and school children, as school busses did not exist. Transport home from the bus stop was conveniently waiting for us when we got off the bus. Now, I realize how kind this lady was to make space available to us, and yet I took it for granted then.

My life was simple. We lived near the English Channel and it was often very windy, forcing us to frequently bike against the wind. If there wasn't rain in the wind, we were content. Today, few children have this independence and life is very different but the habits I developed in childhood, set me up to be independent and athletic, all without a gym membership fee. I was lucky.

The boys' grammar school was about half a mile away from our school, but we never associated with the boys, except for the occasional school dance, to which I was forbidden to go. Each school had about 600 pupils (students) and as these were public schools, everyone got one-third of an Imperial pint of full-cream cow's milk, in a glass bottle, in the middle of the morning, and all but a handful of students had free "school lunches." By choice, Rebecca and I were part of a small group of girls who sat at two tables at the edge of the cafeteria. We ate, what I later learned in America, were called "sack lunches." Why? Because we, along with three others, were vegetarians. No meat for us and only wholegrain bread. Why the other seven or so girls brought sandwiches, is still a mystery. But if Rebecca and I were weird, it didn't worry me, because that was how life was for us. I shrugged it off. Who cared? For sure though, I wasn't going to let anyone know I was bothered by them thinking I was weird!

What did matter to me though, was whether I could run fast, hit a tennis ball hard, shoot hoops well in netball, score runs in rounders and swim well. *Bring it on.* I was up to the challenge. I guess I was born competitive! Without knowing it, Mum set us up to make the most of a healthy lifestyle. We were definitely ahead of the nutritional sciences and exercise programs of our day.

Today, dietary preferences are two-a-penny. If you are entertaining a group of friends at home, it is a good idea to find out if anyone is lactose or gluten intolerant, or perhaps they are allergic to peanuts or strawberries, or are vegans, pesco-vegetarians, or only lacto-ovo-vegetarians. Maybe they choose to eat only GMO-free foods, or need a low-salt diet —or have other dietary restrictions, or preferences. Labeling dishes as vegetarian, or containing pork or shellfish, might be an option too. What a different world we live in! As a consequence of my "weird" childhood, I foolishly never worried that my children would have a serious illness, but thankfully, they didn't.

* * *

Some very young infants are admitted to the PedsICU for "failing to thrive." They can be as young as a few days old, or as old as a few months —but something is wrong. They are not thriving as they should. Very occasionally they are admitted to the floor when they would have had only a few days to live had they not been brought to PedsICU. Once admitted, some require immediate ventilatory support and our Intensivists set about stabilizing and maintaining them, while various pediatric specialists are called in to confirm and treat a suspected diagnosis, or determine an obscure metabolic disorder or syndrome. Multiple diagnostic tests may be ordered which may or may not be run in our hospital's clinical lab. Specialists order some tests that are so obscure that they are performed only occasionally at regional centers and getting results from send-out tests can sometimes take days, or even weeks. The waiting is never easy for parents.

Sydney, a newly diagnosed diabetic, was two-years-old. She was fortunate to be on a life support machine in PICU. *Really? Lucky?* Sydney was lucky because she was alive and, although she would have diabetes for the rest of her life, she was going home. She had not been misdiagnosed, nor medically mismanaged, and her parents had taken action before it was too late. She had made it to the PedsICU in time.

Sydney had been critical for only a few days with atypical symptoms of new-onset diabetes. With no one in her family a diabetic, the thought had never occurred to them. Thankfully, physicians in her community hospital acted on their hunch, knew what to do and sent her to us. In time her family would learn how to manage her diabetes and she could expect to lead a normal life. For Sydney, diabetes would be a way of life that was different from most children around her and her family needed to take her diagnosis seriously. As she grew up, she would not have the absolute freedom that other kids had and failure to comply with certain stipulations sometimes caused immediate problems or later, long-term comorbidities. Disregard of some fundamental guidelines could even be fatal. The PICU saw a few rebellious teens come through our doors as they challenged medical advice, and were rescued, usually. Learning life's lessons is never easy, especially with such high stakes. However, supported by advanced medical science, Sydney could overcome the challenges of being a diabetic, and thrive. Sydney was lucky.

* * *

Cherise was lucky too. When she was born, her initial blood sugar was five, not 35 mg/dl, which is considered the lowest, safe blood-sugar level in a newborn. The Labor and Delivery staff was alarmed. They followed the protocols established for low blood sugars but Cherise's glycemic levels were life-threatening and she was immediately transferred to the out-lying hospital's NICU for initial stabilization. It was a small unit and our Transport Team was soon on the way to bring her to a regional center where she was maintained on life-support. What was causing this severe neonatal hypoglycemia? Something was definitely wrong.

The Pediatric Endocrinologist determined that Cherise was unable to utilize glucose, and that her liver could not store glycogen. It was a rare metabolic condition. This began a lifetime of doctors' appointments, hospitalizations and observation for her young parents. Cherise was an only child, and her parents were fully vested in doing all they could to assist Cherise's pediatricians. Continuous feedings through a nasogastric tube were initiated. Later they were given to her through a gastrostomy tube, and her parents were forced to enter a world they previously knew nothing about. Her mother, a teacher, rose to the occasion and Cherise became a frequent flier when even common childhood illnesses occurred. For her out-patient team of pediatricians, care was trial and error. Cherise was unique, but her parents were grateful she had not become a perinatal mortality statistic. They were ready to learn how to care for their precious daughter.

I last saw Cherise when her proud grandmother flicked through her phone showing me a happy, bright, healthy little 2½-year-old, having fun on the beach. Cherise carried a small backpack containing soy formula on her back. She received feedings continuously through a G-tube. Grandma told me excitedly, "She's going to start eating soon."

Cherise was another success story –a little life saved by modern medicine. Although Cherise will have to learn how to chew and swallow food with the help of Speech Therapists, her strange life is a happy, almost normal one but with countless hurdles ahead of her. The first food she will eat will be determined by her speech therapist, dietician and pediatric endocrinologist! But, having never eaten food in the usual way, she had no desire to eat food like regular kids do –ever. However, her parents (and grandparents) are ready to do what it takes to help their little heroine take the next step in her miracle journey.

More often though, it wasn't a metabolic disease that brought children through our doors, even though new-onset diabetes cases were not uncommon. Our unit admitted many children onto the Pediatric Trauma Service, unfortunately. As a child, I was fortunate in that I was rarely taken to see a physician. Scarlet fever gave my mother a scare, as did a fractured arm when I was four years old and bounced off my bed, but she recovered –and so did I. God must have taken care of me, despite my fool-hardiness.

* * *

Morgan was a lucky kid too.

Good Luck, Bad Luck

Morgan went to a minor league baseball game with his parents, when he was hit on the head by a fly ball. He lost consciousness, but came around quickly. He surely was a lucky three-year-old. His parents were very thankful that he was okay, and they all went home at the end of the game. However, later that evening, Morgan vomited spontaneously and was somnolent. Realizing that something was wrong, they took him to the Peds ER where a simple head X-ray showed a depressed skull fracture, and a head CT showed swelling in the underlying brain tissue. A slow bleed into the brain had caused increased intracranial pressure, and caused the vomiting and drowsiness.

For two days Morgan stayed in the PedsICU for observation. Follow-up diagnostic tests showed that the swelling, and bleeding around his brain, were resolving without any interventions. He made a remarkable recovery and was soon transferred to the Step-down ICU for less intense observation before being discharged home two days later. Being hit on the head by a fly ball and sustaining a skull fracture could have resulted in a much worse injury and outcome. And, had his parents ignored the vomiting, the story would not have had such a happy ending. Yes, Morgan was lucky and his parents realized this.

Pulled muscles, broken bones, grazes, pain and swelling are the lot of being an active kid, but Sean wasn't as lucky as Morgan. In fact, Sean was decidedly unlucky — or perhaps luck had nothing to do with it.

* * *

It was summer time. The season for outdoor fun and craziness, a time for swimming, tree-climbing, cycling, and skateboarding. Fun...fun...fun —until it turns into a nightmare.

Sean's mom, Diedre, heard the kids' screams before she could get out of the shower.

"Sean's fallen out of the tree!"

"He's not moving!"

"Hurry, hurry. Sean's dead."

Sean's frantic seven-year-old playmates, and nine-year-old brother, burst into the house in a quiet, upper-class neighborhood just six miles from the PICU. Diedre's heart missed more than one beat as she grabbed her towel and dialed 911.

"My son's fallen out of a tree...I haven't seen him yet...I was in the shower...He's not moving...Hurry, please."

When she last saw Sean, he and his friends were cycling up and down the cul-de-sac. Now, pulling on clothes over her damp skin, she flew out of the front door almost tripping over kids' bikes strewn in the driveway. She dashed to her son's side.

Sean lay motionless on the sidewalk under a large tree. *Thank God he's breathing. He isn't dead.* Diedre was a nurse who worked in the Out-Patient Surgery Center at a local hospital. She had never been a trauma nurse, but she knew that Sean was still alive, even if severely injured. "Sean! Sean! Mommy's here," she said placing her hand gently on him. "Open your eyes, Sean." He did, and she sighed with relief. He was obeying a simple command.

The neighbors gathered around and Stevie, Sean's brother, stood behind his mom almost paralyzed with fear.

"He fell from way up there, Mom," he said pointing high up into the tree. "I saw it happen...I didn't know he was up there."

The EMS arrived in minutes. They immobilized Sean and secured him to the gurney. With an IV in place, he was red-lighted to the Pediatric ER and eventually admitted to the PedsICU.

Forty-eight hours later, Sean's parents were coming to the realization that their son was a paraplegic. When he hit the ground, Sean had seriously fractured his lumbar spine. It was doubtful that he would be able to use his legs again. It would not be helpful to say to his parents, "Sean is lucky he isn't a quadriplegic," —even though it was true. Sean *was* fortunate that he was not a quad. Being a paraplegic definitely had advantages over being a quadriplegic —or being dead. But for now, that was definitely not a helpful comment.

Stephen, Sean's dad, was extremely distressed.

"How am I going to tell Sean that the life he has always known, is over?" he said as he paused at the Nurses Station. "It's never going to be the same again. He'll never walk or run —or climb trees again."

The fact was there were a lot of things Sean wouldn't be able to do and endless doctor appointments were on the horizon. Sean would face a mountain of challenges. But, on the bright side, being disabled opened up opportunities to him that normal kids could not access. Sean would learn skills normal children never learned and he would forever see life from a different perspective. Perhaps he would be a great swimmer, or even a mountaineer. He could contend for a place in the Special Olympics. He could join a basketball league for wheel-chair users or become a brilliant scientist or physician. Some physicians had even made this incredible career decision while they were kids in PedsICU.

"I don't know how I am going to get us through it all," Stephen said. "It's a disaster." He was totally overwhelmed.

I listened. It was a disaster, but if everyone in Sean's family pulled together, each day could be a small victory.

"I'm sorry it happened," I said. "I will be praying for you all, especially Sean." *What a stupid thing to say. They might be atheists.* But to me, Jesus is the Great Physician and prayer does make a difference. One day, Sean might look back on this accident as being the best thing that happened to him. For sure, I have met many kids with disabled siblings who also rate exceptionally high on character qualities such as compassion, determination, emotional insight and maturity, and respect for others. These qualities are difficult to teach children whose families are seemingly flawless.

Falling from the tree changed Sean's future forever, and no words could convey my feeling of helplessness as I listened to Sean's dad express his sense of failure and fear of the unknown. He was the leader of the household and the family's protector. How could he have let his son, and his whole family, down like this? It wasn't rational, but if he was looking for any consolation, it was that Sean was still alive, which was more than could be said for Justin.

* * *

Justin also fell from a tree, and he fell only 15-feet. Justin was not allowed to climb the tall tree outside his house, he knew that. He was a good climber, and it was fun. *Parents can be spoil-sports!*

Unfortunately Justin's head took the brunt of the fall as it hit the edge of the curb. His skull cracked open partially but, even with some nasty fractures, Justin wasn't killed by the fall, and he too arrived in the PedsICU.

Like Diedre, Justin's mom had known Justin was playing outside as she busied herself with chores. She checked on him through the window as she passed from the kitchen to the living room. He was playing near the tree, but then when she looked out again, she saw no sign of Justin. She went to the door. "Justin?" she yelled.

"Yes Mom," Justin called. "I'm here. I'm in the tree." His mom saw his bare legs among the foliage.

"Get down at once," she yelled, annoyed at him being in the tree. "Don't you dare climb the tree, Justin. Get down now. Do you hear me? Get down. It's dangerous."

"Yes, Mom," Justin said as he climbed a little higher. He heard the front door close. It was exciting being so high —what a great view. He would get down after he'd climbed just a little higher. That was when he made a fatal mistake! He missed his footing and fell to the curb below.

From the start Justin's admission was a roller-coaster for all the staff. I had him for his first three nights. Justin had a large, loving family who made their presence felt right away. They pushed the visitation rules to the limit; they slipped into the unit behind staff or on the tail of other visitors coming through the entrance. They refused to leave the room when asked to, and they argued with the medical and nursing staff over every request made of them. All the while, Justin's condition drifted downwards until the physicians brought his close family into his room, and told them that Justin was brain dead.

Turning in rage, Justin's dad threw a heavy punch through the wall as he screamed profanities in uncontrolled anger. The news was too terrible to hear.

"I told him not to climb the tree," his mom screeched over and over again. "He didn't listen."

Perhaps she was already trying to absolve herself of the blame that she felt.

When the room quietened, our young Attending Physician, Caleb, spoke again. "I am sorry, but I can't bring you any hope."

Caleb was tender-hearted and hated giving such terrible news to any family. The father of two young children, he was committed to saving children's lives. He would never get used to telling parents that their kid would not make it.

"We have done everything we can, but the tests show that he is brain dead. He cannot survive without us breathing for him and keeping his blood pressure up with medicines." Caleb paused. "There is one thing though, that might help you in your grief," Caleb continued. "We are required by law to invite all parents of kids in this condition to consider talking to the Organ Procurement Agency regarding organ donation. It is very likely that many of Justin's organs could be used to save the lives of other children."

Justin's immediate family did not attend church, but they leaned towards donating organs. However, his grandparents were dedicated to their church and strongly opposed organ donation. It wasn't, of course, their decision to make.

Later Justin's mom took me aside and said, "Don't tell my parents we're donating his organs. It would cause a lot of problems in our family."

I wondered how I would keep Justin's final journey to the OR to donate organs a secret from her parents. But, in the end, I didn't need to worry about that because when the Organ Procurement Nurse was finalizing their desire to donate his organs to six or seven (or even more) kids, they changed their minds. He would go to the grave intact. They were not going to donate any of his organs. *Nada.* "Not even his corneas," they said emphatically to the nurse as she left.

Despite the diagnosis, the family continued to demand delays. They wanted another chance, another test, another…whatever was available, despite knowing that Justin was brain dead and would never come back to life.

On the fourth day, Justin's life support was turned off and not one child received a new chance at life through him.

Had Justin obeyed his Mom and not climbed the tree, there would be no story to tell. But all too often kids copy the behaviors they see modeled in their homes. Justin mimicked what he saw. He was doing things his own way, just like they did. Why should he obey their rules when they pushed the limits and fiercely argued against the requests of others? Lying was convenient, especially if it served their purpose; rules were unjust and troublesome —so they attempted to circumvent them. What was a very sad admission in the first place, was made worse for the staff by a difficult, non-compliant family. Sadly, Justin had learned disobedience and defiance from his family, but in disobeying the home rules, he lost his life.

The question remains, was Justin's death an accident? Some would say, "Yes, it was a tragic accident. He was very unlucky." Others give a resounding, "No, it was an unfortunate consequence."

Whatever it was, death was too high a price to pay for disobedience, or for learning well from misguided parents. It is unlikely that Justin's family ever saw his death as anything other than a terrible accident. It is unlikely that they would change their parenting strategies as a result of Justin's death. But to the Team, it was a bad, sad story, where everyone was a loser —Justin, his family, the children still waiting for a new chance in life, and their families too.

CHAPTER 5

Jack Fell Down...

LIKE MOST CHILDREN who grow up in the countryside, I endured my fair share of cuts and scrapes. Falling off my bicycle, tripping when skipping, slipping in the mud and landing short of the other side of the channels that crisscrossed the marshlands where we walked our dogs. No serious falls —except for the fractured humerus when I was four. I had been told not to bounce on my bed, but bouncing was fun.

As I grew older, I thought that serious accidents did not happen to law-abiding citizens living in my little corner of the UK. If you could swim, you would never drown. If you could ride a bike, cars would never hit you as long as you kept to the side. It was your fault if you stabbed yourself with scissors when you were running, so don't run with scissors.

In my teens, as the summer holidays dragged on, Rebecca and I thought nothing of bicycling three miles to the beach to swim. We biked through our village, down a hill, through a farm and along a mile of grassy track that ran through marshland. We then lifted our bicycles over a 5-bar gate, checked (both ways) for the high-speed electric trains that ran between London and Ramsgate, and, if clear, crossed the double track. After heaving our bikes over the next 5-bar gate, we pedaled a short distance along a gravel path to the beach –which we usually had to ourselves. We swam in the cold English Channel for as long as we could tolerate it, hoping that the sun would come out for a while and stop us from shivering. Pulling our clothes on over sticky, salty bodies, we hobbled back up the pebbly beach, to bike home again. That activity took care of a whole afternoon. We never drowned, nor were we washed over to France on the small inflated air-mattresses that we stashed on the back of our bikes. We stuck bicycle tire tube patches on holes in the inflatable mattresses and had a lot of fun. But safe? *Of course, it was safe.* We even swam among a swarm of harmless, translucent, white jelly-fish which slapped our arms and legs as we swam. The solution? Swim harder and you didn't feel them. It was part of the adventure. Today, I would think twice about swimming in those frigid seas, and would definitely not let my children, or grandchildren, live such reckless lives!

Although my mother considered me a dimwit, I guess I wasn't because at 12-years-old I joined my sister at Simon Langton Grammar School for Girls in Canterbury. We wore school uniforms, studied hard (at least Rebecca did) and played netball (like basketball for girls only, but with no ball-bouncing or backboard on the hoop), badminton, table tennis and hockey –field hockey, between September and April. In the summer term, rounders (a game like under-arm baseball), tennis and athletics (track and field) were our choices. We swam in an outdoor pool when the water was over 60° F. Today, athletes are encouraged to wear wetsuits when racing in 60° F water –but it was invigorating, if not horribly cold, but I loved sports.

For the first two years my class was seated alphabetically, so I got a front row seat, beside the door. Selina Baker was three rows to my left, and three seats back. After the Easter holidays, she returned to school sporting a golden tan and told us fascinating stories of skiing in the Swiss Alps. It sounded brilliant, but I could only imagine it —like most of us. Skiing was for rich kids, which cut me out, and, living in southern England meant that snow fell on only a few days each winter, consequently I didn't ski.

But 45 years later, I decided I'd learn to ski in the Cascade Mountains in Oregon. I mastered the bunny-slopes —just, but later I was half-way down a mid-sized slope when I fell, and slid another 20-feet, stopping in soft snow at the edge of the ski run. I lay off to the side holding my right arm to my body. My shoulder was so painful that I could not move my arm an inch. My husband came and stood a little downhill from me with his pole extended towards me.

"Grab on," he said. "I'll help you up." But I couldn't get up. So he came around and pushed me up from behind onto my skis, and started winding backwards down the slope in front of me. Not being the best of downhill skiers, and having skied this slope only a few times before, getting down to the lodge was a long, slow journey.

My skiing fall wasn't a classic GLF, but x-rays showed a chipped shoulder, which was painful enough. It happened in seconds and curbed my desire to down-hill ski. Perhaps I should leave skiing to Selena, and my husband, and just snow-shoe in the great outdoors of the north-west.

Southern California outdoorsmen, or women, can pick and choose their sport while living in comparative comfort. It is sheer paradise. In winter, one can spend a day skiing or snowboarding, if that is your skill-set, at a nearby ski resort and return, exhausted, to the warm sunshine of the valley in less than two hours. Alternatively, one can drive two hours along crowded freeways to play beach volleyball, take a swim or read a good book on the beach while getting a perfect tan. By late evening, one is home again, invigorated, tanned and happy. A ninety-minute drive west could land one in the desert where the terrain is dotted with Joshua trees and lends itself to photography, hiking, and relaxing in tee-shirt and shorts. As the sun drops behind giant boulders, one can cozy-up to a crackling camp fire and gaze at millions of stars shining through black velvet skies above, as the temperatures fall. So relaxing. So incredible.

Working at IVCH allowed me to enjoy the outdoors, and I did.

Brits are known for their prowess in sitting sports like cycling, riding (horse-back riding) and canoeing. You can confirm this when watching the Summer Olympics, however I rode poorly. My mother's photo albums displayed photos of my older sisters winning trophies at gymkhanas, long before I was born, but by the time I came along, the coffers were empty, and Rebecca and I rode bicycles, not horses. With little extra money, riding lessons didn't last for long, and they did not prepare me for the wild ride I went on as a nursing student. Galloping through open fields with a nurse-friend, an excitable 14-hand horse tossed me off and I found myself looking up into my friend's face against a backdrop of grey clouds —only to lose consciousness again. The next day I woke up in the dorm with a sore head and no recollection of how my friend and her mother had gotten me home. Concussion? Yes. Thankfully I was wearing a riding hat, but where did that day go? What did my CT scan show? How were my neuro checks? Thanks to God's watch-care I survived, and of course CT scanners did not exist then. But in PICU, not all falls are GLFs either, nor from horses or beds —and not everything can be mended, like my arm —twice. For all my escapades, though, I had a relatively incident-free life, even avoiding common injuries at work over a long nursing career.

Long before the term "Incident Report Form" was coined, nurses taped one-inch metal files to their scissors to cut through tough glass ampoules of medication. Occasionally, one accidentally nicked oneself on an inadequately sawn-off vial while cracking the top off. *Oh well.* Once I incurred a rather deep cut on my left thumb doing just that. It needed stitches but I applied pressure after checking for shards of glass, and slapped on some gauze under a tight bandage. That did the trick. No need to go to the ER, or document the occurrence. I still have the scar to show for it!

* * *

In the PICU staff catch glimpses of the price some kids pay for their foolish, but often innocent actions, or for having parents who are too busy to keep track of them. Parents can be distracted by social media, too many things going on around them, complicated schedules and the like, or they ignore dangers that would warn them of an accident ready to happen right in front of their eyes had they been looking. Some take drugs —but that's another story. Other parents are fully involved with their child's activities, but — for one split second they turn away. Too late. The damage has occurred, and no one can turn the clock back for even one moment.

Sadly, the PICU staff is all too familiar with scenarios where innocent games turn into disasters. Swimming with friends becomes a drowning, or near-drowning incident (and many PICU nurses are of the opinion that near-drowning can be worse than drowning, when it comes to the long-term consequences). Careless cycling can result in irreparable head injuries. Snowboarding ends up as an accidental death, and swinging from a tree turns into a hanging, or maybe a 20-foot fall onto the bare ground below. It happens. Falling from all sorts of places brings kids into PICU, sometimes in a grave condition.

* * *

Jessica was 18-months-old when she fell through the screen window from a second-floor apartment, onto the dirt below. Her life was probably saved by her encountering a small bush just before hitting the packed dirt. Nevertheless, she found her way to the PICU through an Emergency Room in a small community hospital out in the desert. She was transported by ground for a "higher level of care" after our Attending received the referring ER doc's report. The Transport Team was greeted eagerly by the ER staff.

"We're so glad you're here. Come this way."

Dutifully following directions, the Team and I wound our way past waiting patients, and then bays filled with big people who had come to the ER to find treatment for their ailments. We continued on to the only kid in the ER —and her apprehensive parents.

"Looking after little kids is very scary," the anxious nurse said to me. "I hope everything is alright. We don't get many critical peds here, you know."

Everything was usually fine. Most ERs did a great job with the resources they had, and today was no exception. The nurse reported off to me while the ER doc updated our PICU Resident. Jessica was neurologically fine. No serious head injury, thank God. The RT checked the respiratory status of our newest little charge. I checked the IV infusion, and changed it to follow our doctor's new orders, and gave the stat meds ordered. Jessica was stable and very fortunate. Her guardian angel must have been watching over her as she fell. But where was that angel before she fell? With his back turned, like Jessica's mother? But that is another question.

We attached Jessica to our monitors, as the worried parents talked to the physician, half wanting to detain him with more questions, but mindful of the need for their kid to leave for the PICU. They signed the consent form for us to provide treatment for Jessica and then, like a well-oiled machine, with everyone doing their part to expedite getting the kid loaded, and on the way, we swept into action and left.

Jessica was fortunate. The Pediatric Neurosurgeons worked with our Intensivist. A head CT revealed no severe soft-tissue injuries and no significant bleeding into the brain. The abdominothoracic CT was negative too. Amazingly she had no broken bones anywhere. *Praise God for the bush that saved her life.*

Jessica stayed in PedsICU a few days. IV fluids, 12-hours of intensive neurological observation in the PICU, antibiotic ointment to grazes, and an appointment-cum-lecture for her parents the next day from the Safe Kids Coalition Team on how to avoid accidents at home, filled her stay with us. After 24-hours on the floor she was transferred to the Step-down ICU. Jessica would have follow-up care with her own pediatrician once she was home.

Jessica was lucky, really lucky. And perhaps the scare taught her parents a life-saving lesson that they would have never learned without that frightening occurrence.

Many children, like Jessica, pass through PICU quickly. Kids like to climb, and with their cerebral cortices not fully developed, they do some silly, dangerous things. I did. Not recognizing the probable consequences of their actions, nor the dangers, nor being justifiably fearful or careful, nasty accidents can happen –but climbing is fun! Rocks, hillsides, play-ground equipment, garage roofs, ladders, and trees are all fair game. Trees are especially versatile. They are climbable, can be swung on and jumped off. Kids hide in them and behind them. So much fun! And water? That's fun too. It is not just for taking a shower in or drinking. It's for splashing in, jumping and diving into, jet skiing on and swimming in. Water is so enticing –and yet dangerous. Parents often have childhood memories of safely climbing trees, diving into and swimming in lakes and rivers near their homes on stiflingly hot summer days — and nothing terrible happened. Today, things look different. Accidents happen, and local TV channels and social media are on hand to inform the world of tragic goings-on. But, let's forget that, we say. It doesn't happen to our kids. Unfortunately, the PICU staff knows differently. Dave, like Jessica, fell, but his fall had a whole different outcome.

Dave was 15, and had also fallen from the second floor, from the balcony onto the dirt below. The difference was that he weighed a lot more than did Jessica, and no bush broke his fall. Consequently, his injuries were much worse. Like many teens who think it's cool to perform death-defying feats and post them on YouTube for notoriety and fame, Dave was into risky behaviors. However, like many kids his age, he didn't realize that actions had consequences –sometimes dire consequences.

While his parents were out for the evening, Dave got drunk at a friend's house (first mistake) and fell off the balcony (second mistake). He was brought directly to our Peds ER by ambulance, with severe head injuries. Time was of essence. Peds Neurosurgery was notified and they wasted no time in getting Dave into OR to prevent further brain injury. Dave was admitted to the Peds ICU after his surgery. He had a ventricular drain in place, and a bolt to monitor pressures inside his brain. Dave was intubated and sedated, but not so heavily as to camouflage any neurological changes. I was working the day shift when I caught up with Dave for the first time. He had been with us for almost 24-hours.

His nurse, Jim, had Dave as a one-to-one and it was almost the end of a hectic shift. Jim still hadn't given Dave his bed bath, or changed his bed linen, something Jim should do before the night shift arrived. He did most of the bed bath before calling in reinforcements: an RT and four extra nurses. We stood around Dave's bed, ready for action.

"Okay guys," Jim announced. "We're a team and need to be quick. Katie, you're in charge of the airway and ventilator. Okay?" *Good choice —Katie was an RT and the best for that job.* "You two guys," he said pointing towards two nurses standing near the door, "You go on the left side of the bed and keep control over there. Remember, he's got 4-point restraints, but who knows what will happen? Tabitha, you take his feet —and don't take the restraints off before you have to. *As if I would!* Ciera, you do the sheets after I wash his back." We stationed ourselves as instructed and checked Dave's lines for movability. We were ready for action. "I've bumped up his sedation, but watch out," Jim said, "he's feisty."

Dave was big and strong. We would release Dave's hands and feet in sequence, roll him, bathe his back, put in new linen and roll him again, all the while hanging onto his lines and tubings. It would take a matter of minutes to bathe him and change his bed, if we followed the plan.

"Let's roll," Jim said. And we did, but within seconds of my releasing Dave's right foot, it shot out at Frances and struck her squarely on the chest. She lost her balance and fell out of sight, onto the floor. I grabbed the restraint which was still attached to the wayward foot, and frantically wound it around my hand, pulling it tight. Immediately Frances popped up.

"You okay, Fran?" Jim asked. "Want to fill out an incident report?"

Fran grinned.

"I'm fine," she said, "and no. I've documented enough today thank you very much!"

Three minutes later, Dave was again fully restrained. We had bumped-up the sedation even further, and it took effect. He lay immobile on a clean bed. I filed out behind Frances. "I'm sorry, Fran...He was so quick...I don't know how it happened."

Tender-hearted Fran listened.

"It happens to the best of us, Tabitha. He's a big guy and his head is so messed up, we should have had an RT and *six* extra nurses, not four." She went on. "Jim's had a rough shift dealing with Dave's agitation. I'll be surprised if the kid is problem-free neuro-wise, in a year."

It was three whole weeks before Dave was ready for transfer to the Step-down Unit. During this time, I cared for him on a few shifts. On transfer though, like many neuro kids, Dave was still occasionally aggressive and unwieldy and had both short and long-term memory deficits. But he could answer simple, direct questions, and no longer needed to stay in PedsICU.

Two weeks after his transfer off our floor, I happened to be on Station One when I saw a kid being pushed in a wheelchair onto the unit. "Tabitha?" the woman behind the wheelchair called out. Hearing my name, I stopped and looked intently at the figure down the hallway. Dave's mom? *Drat, my eyesight.* She carried on towards the desk. Sure enough, Dave's mom had wheeled him over to see the PedsICU nurses. I gave her a quick hug.

"So how's he doing, Mom?" A simple, effective way to address a patient's mother when you have forgotten their name. "What's Dave doing now?" Apparently he wasn't walking, but he surely must be a whole lot better.

"Oh, he's getting on super," she answered. Dave stared straight ahead, seemingly unaware of where he was. I got down to his level, and put my hand on his shoulder.

"Hi, Dave. You look a lot better than when I last saw you," —which was the truth. "How are you feeling?" Dave said nothing.

"Your scars look great," I continued enthusiastically. "And your hair is growing back. Wonderful. Any headaches?"

No reply.

"Dave, honey," his mother interjected. "Do you have a headache?" Pause. "You do remember being here, don't you?" No answer. "This is Tabitha," she continued. "She looked after you a number of times when you were here." Another blank stare.

Seemingly embarrassed by Dave's lack of response, she told the admiring group of nurses that Dave was now eating by himself and could walk a little. He was getting intensive physical therapy which helped him a great deal. "Every day he's doing something new," she said brightly. Then bending down to Dave's ear, she said, "We're going to see Jim now, Dave. You must remember Jim."

We gave her directions to where Jim was, and she wheeled him off towards Station Three. I felt sorry for Dave's mom after his disappointing performance.

A while later, Dave's mom wheeled him back towards the exit. I caught up with them as they went towards the locked doors, to help them get out. "How did it go? Did Dave remember Jim?" I quietly asked as we walked along.

Her crestfallen appearance, and Dave's empty stares, told me the answer.

"He didn't remember anyone," Mom said. "I couldn't get him to remember anything." She wiped a tear quickly from her eye as I held the door open for them to go through. Putting my hand on her shoulder, I said, "I'll be praying for you both. It's got to be rough for you. It's going to be a long haul –but he's come a long way already." Dave's mom smiled weakly. It was the truth if you compared how he was now with how he was when we admitted him to the floor. But the old Dave had gone, and perhaps would never reappear, at least not for a very long time.

I never learned as to what extent Dave recovered. Head injury patients take months, or even years to recover, rather than days and weeks. Their family's active involvement in their recovery, and the kid's fundamental personality, factor into the degree of improvement attained. If Dave never fully recovered from his fall, it was a heavy price to pay for two bad choices. But parents cannot be wholly responsible for a kid's accident when the kid is 15.

However, was Dave's fall an accident or the consequence of poor choices mixed with defiance, immaturity, and alcohol? That mix can be lethal to kids and adults alike, and has the habit of catching up with them sooner, rather than later. Dave's sad story reminded me of how blessed I was to have three healthy kids.

* * *

Skyler was just 2-months-old when his mom, Diane, took him to a baseball game. It was an excellent way for the family to spend an evening. His older brother had signed up to play baseball in the rec league, and the weather was beautiful. The summer sun hung over the horizon as the games proceeded, and cheers echoed across the field as players dove for balls and lunged at pitches.

"Hustle, Kyler," Diane yelled. She cheered and clapped as he played like a future league player. Chatting to the parents around her, she sipped her iced soda. It was a warm, summer evening. Skyler slept quietly next to Diane, strapped in his car seat on the bleachers, oblivious to the noises erupting around him. The floodlights came on as the deep orange-red globe dipped out of sight, enveloping the spectators in warm darkness. A spectacular evening for a ball game in southern California.

Kyler's game was exciting. The lead changed hands several times, and outstanding defensive plays studded a great game. By the ninth inning, Kyler's team was still down three runs when one of his team-mates hit a grand slam, giving the team a dramatic come-from-behind win. The crowd went wild, exploding into cheers and, standing with one accord, they moved the bleachers just enough to cause Skyler to fall through them, still strapped in his seat, onto the concrete 10-feet below. Diane screamed as she saw him go, but was unable to stop him.

"My baby!" she yelled —and Skyler's head hit the concrete with a thud.

Confusion and panic set in as Diane tore to the end of the bleachers screaming hysterically, and bounded down the steps towards the field. Her screams alerted others who saw the accident. A couple of bystanders scrambled under the bleachers to reach Skyler's limp body before she got to him. He was still strapped in his car seat, and silent. He looked dead.

Paramedics rushed Skyler at break-neck speed to the Peds ER, and before more than a few minutes had passed, Skyler was in OR where the Pediatric Neurosurgeons were waiting for him. Not a minute would be lost.

When Skyler arrived in the PedsICU, his swollen head that had previously felt like a well-cracked, hard-boiled egg, was securely hidden under layers of bandages. Two small collapsed drainage bulbs dangled like weights from beneath what looked like a mound of snow —his head dressing. He was quiet, subdued by the surgery, and to some measure, by the sedation he was receiving for comfort.

With the fall, Skyler had bled into his brain and under his bruised scalp, and, adding to that, the surgery has resulted in his face swelling so that he was almost beyond recognition. He sat strapped in yet another car seat, one of ours this time. The seat was safely secured inside the crib, to the rails. The crib rails were up. There was no chance he would fall anywhere. His head was elevated and steadied to decrease the risk of increasing intercranial pressure and unnecessary movement.

Diane sat in the recliner a few feet from him watching his every breath and listening to the monitors clicking reassuringly. Guilt hammered through her mind. Now, with twenty-twenty hindsight, she realized she could have avoided the accident if Skyler had been strapped to her body in a baby sling, and not in the car seat. She could have skipped going to the game, but she had wanted to be there for Kyler, but the thought of such a terrible accident happening, had never entered her mind.

One of the benefits of Skyler being only two-months-old was that his skull was comparatively soft and his cranium had shattered into small pieces, loosely tied together by his scalp. This allowed his head to swell without causing too much serious damage to his brain inside his skull. This was a real blessing, and over the next few days the external swelling subsided and Diane began to see Skyler's familiar little face emerge from under the layers of bandages.

Just one week later I pushed Skyler's crib out of the unit. Mylar balloons drifted above him as we made our way down the interior hall towards the Step-down ICU. There were so many "get-well" inflatables that his crib almost seemed to fly. Skyler sat in his seat amid an ocean of cuddly toys sprawled around the crib and peeking through the bars. His eyes were glued to the fluorescent lights as we rolled along. Diane followed the entourage smiling broadly.

"This must have been some journey for you, Diane," I said. She nodded. "And Skyler's recovering extremely fast. That is wonderful." We swung a right and headed for the door. "How are *you* doing, Diane?" I asked. "This week must've been a nightmare."

How our parent's deal with their emergency is impossible to know as each situation is unique, but few endure less than sky-rocketing stress on our floor. Diane nodded her head again.

"Yes, we've prayed a lot for Skyler —and all of you. Our team of doctors and nurses have been amazing. We know He's in control," she said, pointing up towards the ceiling.

"I believe that too, Diane. I can tell you a few stories about God visiting the PICU for real." I paused. "Skyler's got his appetite back too," I said. "I must remember to document that 6-ounce bottle he demolished just before we left the floor!"

Diane smiled again. It was good to hear another parent speak with faith in the Great Physician. Despite what I see every day, I still know God's in control. Research shows that faith in God makes a huge difference when life takes a downturn —even when death snatches a kid away. Our extremity *is* God's opportunity.

Later I heard through the grape-vine that Skyler spent two weeks in the Step-down ICU and then went to Basic Peds before he was discharged home. For the Team, Skyler's PICU admission and week's stay was a success story and had Diane on cloud nine when Skyler was transferred off the floor. As to how Skyler fared in the long run, I have no clue. Brain injury recovery is a long journey for most patients, and an uncertain journey. Diane's faith would be tested over months, and perhaps even over many years. Who could tell? Perhaps Skyler would develop seizures, or experience severe headaches. Would his mother's innocent mistake impact his whole life? No one knew.

The fact is little kids are vulnerable and at the mercy of their parent's common sense. Accidents can be avoided if we knew what was around each corner, but that is an impossible dream. It is so easy to miss an invisible warning! But Safe Practice Policies are developed for health care institutions so that in-house errors are avoided and could be important for the home environment too. PICU nurses know that.

* * *

After my miniscule shoulder injury from skiing, I struggled with deep pain for months. Steroid injections decreased it and improved my shoulder function, and physical therapists taught me exercise regimens which I repeated every day. I plastered print-outs of the exercises on my refrigerator so that I didn't get sloppy in doing my work-outs, and slowly my shoulder healed, almost entirely. I was blessed by having only a shoulder injury.

An incredible Creator fearfully and wonderfully made us, but injuries occur in a flash, and repair may take months or years, or never happen. Skyler's head mended miraculously, making us optimistic about his future. I believe God worked through the hands of gifted surgeons and a Team of professionals who expect, and often see, miracles happen in PedsICU.

CHAPTER 6

Wake Up, Son

MY EARLIEST CHILDHOOD MEMORIES always included action. Playing ball, swimming, roller skating. I loved to compete –and win. Sports were serious business to me, so I missed out on playing sports for the fun of it. I played to win, and when I didn't, I had to learn to lose graciously. Now that was difficult! I still enjoy participating in road races and triathlons, and still do my best to pass someone, anyone, in front of me. One of my kids is also competitive. I wonder how that happened! So, when a strong, athletic kid becomes ill, I take notice. It is a little too close to me for comfort.

* * *

Homero was a kid who left his own prints on my heart. Some kids do that. His was a particularly devastating case, not because I built a strong relationship with him or his family, but because his admission was extraordinarily intense and unforgettable. How did an athletic Hispanic kid die in less than 24-hours of coming to PedsICU?

I was on a three-in-a-row schedule and was ready for a challenge on my first night. The assignments were handed out and, as luck would have it, I got the new admit. "Here's to a great night," I said as I picked up the beige assignment card and grabbed my stuff off the table. Walking to the far end of the unit, I turned into Station Three, and was ready for report at the bedside. Homero looked pretty good. A handsome guy too. But looks can be deceptive —and they were.

Homero was a strong 15-year-old Hispanic kid. He had been admitted to PedsICU in the middle of the afternoon. He was unusually pale, but any mother would be exceedingly proud of a son like Homero, and his mother was. According to the report, Homero was a keen soccer player. That struck a chord in me. As transplanted-Brits, my family and I tried to keep up with the English Football League, especially Premiere Division games. A few days earlier Homero had scored the winning goal in a friendly game at school, and yet he looked sturdy enough to become a line-backer in a few years. That was what made his illness so curious. He was a healthy, seemingly strong kid doing regular stuff up to being admitted, and yet he was always tired. In retrospect though, his striking frame and youthful energy had covered up the evidence of an insidious disease that a frailer, less energetic kid may have complained about sooner.

Eventually, Homero's mom and dad took him to the doctor to find the cause for his tiredness. They found their answer. Homero's hemoglobin was 3.6mg/dl. *No wonder he was tired. It was exceedingly low.* The doctor sent him immediately to our Peds ER at Inland Valley Children's Hospital for more blood tests. The journey took almost two hours to drive. The lab results indicated that Homero had AML, acute myelogenous leukemia, and because of the severity of his illness, the docs admitted Homero immediately for intensive treatment and observation in the PICU. That afternoon he came by gurney to the floor, stepped onto the standing-scales to be weighed, and then got into bed. His nurse hooked him up to the monitors and admitted him just as she would any other kid –vital signs, initial strip from the cardiac monitor, and chit-chat about likes and dislikes. Homero didn't care though. He was too exhausted to worry about anything.

"I bet he'll be snapped up by the NFL in a few years," I predicted as I sat down on the swivel seat and pulled myself towards the counter to get report.

Homero was a one-to-one for the night. It was best to be inside his room for report, just in case something happened, even though his mom was at the bedside. She did not understand English but usually families had to leave the room at report time. However, Homero had been admitted very recently, so Melissa allowed her to stay in the room. The report wouldn't take long.

"What's up with our guy?" I asked Melissa as I settled on the seat, report sheet at the ready. Homero had been in the room a little over an hour and everything had gone well so far.

In ten minutes, the report was finished.

"You have a good night, Tabitha," Melissa said. "I'll see you in the morning."

She picked up her pens and stethoscope, and paused at the door, "If I've forgotten something, let me know tomorrow. I'll do it in the morning," she said.

"Uh-huh," I grunted.

"And don't work too hard," Melissa joked as she disappeared down the hall.

Homero lay motionless on the bed. His mom, a small, grebe woman, was perched on the edge of the recliner, leaning towards him with her hand placed tentatively on his arm as if she wasn't sure if she should touch him. She stared into his face, hoping that he would open his eyes, and that the nightmare would be over. Worn out, Homero was sleeping peacefully. His dad came in after a while. He was a field laborer, and despite his diminutive size, he was the head of the family. Homero was already much taller than his dad who stood quietly beside his wife, touching Homero from time to time.

While things were calm, I got on with the routine tasks of assessing him, checking the doctor's orders and medication times. The monitors clicked in the background. All was quiet. *I'm not going to tell them that only one parent can stay for the night…They've been through a lot today, and it is just the beginning of a very long journey for leukemia. AML isn't a kid-glove disease.* Besides that, my Spanish was limited –limited to asking my patients how they were, what their pain level was and if they are hungry or thirsty.

Perhaps Homero's parents will go home for the night, I thought, *when they are sure that everything's going smoothly. I'll wait. At least they can see that the night nurse is a mature, seasoned nurse!* They could check that one off their list of worries!

In a while, the secretary called into the room over the intercom. "Can Homero's sister come back, Tabitha?"

"Sure. His parents are at the bedside but maybe she's bi-lingual. Have her come back. Thanks."

Rosa was bilingual, much older than Homero and a pre-nursing, college student. She could translate for her parents, and I would be able to provide the answers I needed to complete Homero's database –any previous illnesses, if he was taking any medicines, etc. I didn't call for an in-house translator because Rosa was comfortable answering all my questions, translating medical terms, and telling her parents what was the immediate plan for Homero. Rosa's boy-friend remained in the Visitor's Lounge, and Homero's other sister was on her way to the hospital. She would arrive in a few hours.

Rosa formulated questions for her parents who were shell-shocked, and could not verbalize their concerns to doctors who appeared to be far-removed from their simple lives.

"I will try and get an update on Homero's condition for you from Kirk, one of our Senior Residents," I said. "He will answer your questions."

Kirk, a fourth year Pediatric Resident Physician, discussed Homero's diagnostic reports and immediate care, often referring to his scribbled progress notes. He said that Homero's condition was very critical and that the Team had determined that Homero would do best if he were to rest entirely. That meant that Homero would be intubated, and attached to a breathing machine, a ventilator. Although shocked by this information, Rosa relayed it back to her parents like a pro as I worked in the background.

. I slipped in and out of the room collecting medications and equipment needed for the intubation as his parents learned that Homero would be put into a type of coma to keep him comfortable. They became more unsettled because they could not fully comprehend what was really going on, even though they ultimately wanted what was best for their youngest child.

"He's so strong ... and young. He was playing soccer only last week. Surely the tiredness is only a passing phase," they pled.

Rosa and Dr. Kirk went back and forth, explaining over and over again what the Team considered to be in Homero's best interest. I left the room and Kirk wrote the sedation and intubation orders. I called Homero's RT, giving him an update. Within minutes the RT had a ventilator standing outside the room, ready for use. Rosa then left the room to talk to Kirk.

"My parents want Homero to get the best medical care possible, and if this is what has to be done, they're not going to stand in the way," she reported. "But you can see they are very upset."

Kirk could see that.

The family talked together for a while, and, after signing the informed consent forms, Homero's mom gave him a quick kiss and left the room, her tiny figure supported between two slightly taller, stronger people: her husband and her daughter. As they turned to go down the long hallway to the front of the unit, I heard her sobs and saw her dabbing her eyes with a tissue. Homero's mom looked devastated -and very fragile.

Within 20 minutes, Homero's family was back. Seeing their young, athletic son lying so unfamiliarly attached to the ventilator amidst a maze of intravenous lines and tubes, horrified them. Hadn't they taken him to the doctor for a check-up just this morning? And now? Now they were dealing with words like "leukemia," "critical" and "unconscious"? Words they had never heard before rang in their ears, confusing them so much that they were unable to unscramble their thoughts. Homero's mom stared at him, fumbling with a tissue and hanging onto her husband's arm.

"It's like Homero in a deep sleep," I explained. "He won't remember all of this when he wakes up...The medicine is keeping him comfortable. His heart rate is slower now," I said pointing towards the monitor. "That means he is resting better." They were reassured a little, and whispered among themselves.

I noticed the list of orders growing longer every time I checked Homero's chart. Homero had already received a unit of whole blood, and more was being ordered. Different IV fluids still needed to be hung, and there was lab work scheduled for every two to four hours.

As time passed, the family took turns walking in and out of his room, always anxious. They asked questions through Rosa and stood quietly staring at Homero as I kept on task. The room cleared occasionally when the family retreated to the waiting room, but the orders kept coming, and I felt swamped. Overwhelmed, I paged the Charge Nurse over-head.

Ding...dong. It connected right away.

"Bernie, could you spare me half an hour? I need an extra hand. It's very busy...I'm sinking."

Bernie was at Station Four when he returned my call, and came to Room 14 in an instant. A slim, experienced Charge Nurse in his late thirties, Bernie had gotten out of a lengthy shift report on the 24-patients on the floor only a few minutes earlier, and was making his way around the unit. Starting on Station Five, he was checking on how things were going, who needed help and who was doing fine.

"I knew you'd be calling me," he said as he entered the door. "I was trying to get around everyone else first, because I knew that once I got here, there would be no leaving. So Tabitha, what's up? What can I do?"

"Thanks for coming, Bernie," I said, and started reeling off tasks one by one. "First of all, can you call the Blood Bank and see if Homero's second unit is ready and then, be a sport, and get it for me, please? And then," I continued, "as you go by the desk, check with Connie and see what's up with the x-ray guy. I called the tech 15-minutes ago and he's still not here. Homero was intubated a while ago and…" I was about to continue, when Bernie interrupted me.

"Okay, okay, Tabitha," he said. "I've got the picture. I'll check with the Blood Bank first, and see what's up. Did you send the blood release form?"

"Yes, I did," I said sharply, my temper already a little frayed. "Of course, I did."

"I was just checking," Bernie said. "Cool it, Tabitha, we have a long night ahead. You know how fussy they are down there."

He proceeded to sign in on the computer and check for the blood availability as the rumble of the X-ray machine sounded in the distance.

"The blood looks like it's ready," Bernie said. "I'll take copies of the order, the consent and stickers with me, just in case. You never know what they'll want these days."

He turned to leave as the x-ray tech pushed his way into the room.

"Oh Bernie," I said quickly, "hold it a moment…Give me a hand here first. I sure don't want to extubate Homero accidentally."

I turned to Rosa, who was anxiously watching what was going on and listening to our conversation.

"I'm sorry, but you guys will have to step out for a few minutes so that we can take the x-ray. Could you let your parents know that please, Rosa?"

Everyone shuffled out as Bernie and I heaved Homero onto the x-ray plate and then made a quick exit ourselves, returning to pull the plate out from underneath him a few seconds later. We settled Homero carefully as the x-ray machine rumbled out of the room, and Homero's family came back in.

"Okay, Tabitha. I'm off." Bernie said. "I'll get the blood."

When Bernie came back with the blood, he checked it with me and then I hung it. We both then worked on the doctor's orders that kept coming, and coming, and coming. After what seemed like a very long time, but was little more than an hour and a half, the pace began to slow. The list of orders was manageable once again.

"Well, Tabitha," Bernie said, "I think I'll go now. I haven't been around the unit yet tonight. You'll be okay, won't you?"

"Sure, Bernie...and thanks a lot. It was a scramble, but I'll be okay now. Thanks."

Bernie went out onto the floor leaving me with the family. I sat on the high-stool by the nursing supplies, watching the monitors, IVs, and medications, and documenting Homero's progress.

"I am so sorry that I have been ignoring you guys," I said looking up at Homero's mother and Rosa. "As you know, Homero has been keeping us busy. But things are slowing down now, and he's looking pretty good."

To me, things did look good, but probably no family in their right mind would agree with me. Having your kid lying motionless on the bed, with a breathing tube stuck down his throat, plastic tubing and wires running all over the place, numerous medicines hanging from poles, and blood being pumped in, could hardly be described as "looking good" to any sane person —so I decided to rephrase what I said.

"Well, what I mean is that Homero is stable at the moment, and we have everything on board that he needs right now." *Not exactly a scientific explanation —but it would get the message over, and make them feel more at ease.* "I am very hopeful that things will go smoothly tonight now that he is resting and comfortable," I continued. "You do understand that when he wakes up, he won't recollect anything that has happened to him over the last few hours, don't you? He wasn't in pain when we placed the tube down his airway, and he is resting comfortably."

I tried to put Homero's family at ease, but their shocked expressions gave me little hope that I was successful. *They're probably in mental overload and unable to absorb anything more.* However, knowing they would be leaving for home soon, I pressed on, telling Homero's sister what I expected would happen that night, the medications he would be given, how we were monitoring his vital signs carefully, and that he would rest peacefully.

I charted vital signs and attended to the IVs and medications as the monitors clicked in the background and went around the bed, and from side to side, working busily. The family sat in silence beside Homero's bed, trying to keep out of the way. At times Homero's mom got up and patted his arm gingerly, and then resettled herself on the edge of the seat. The RT joined me, and we suctioned

Homero as the family sat in silence, blindly watching the strange goings-on.

All at once I noticed that Rosa was missing. She had left her forlorn parents sitting on their own. Within minutes the intercom rang out, *ding-dong*, "Tabitha, can you take another in your room? Another sister is here."

"It's a squash," I replied, "–but send her back for a while…we'll manage…It's quiet here now."

Homero's eldest sister rushed into the room and dropped to her knees beside her little brother and hugged him, ignoring the tubes and cables. A little taller than their dad, she draped her arms over her brother's chest and burst into loud sobs, overwhelmed by the prolonged anxiety and relieved to be beside her brother at last. The weekend before, she had watched him playing soccer, and now her little brother lay chemically paralyzed, deathly pale and unconscious in an ICU. It was too much for her, and she sobbed uncontrollably. I looked at the family anxiously. I did not really want to be distracted by the family's goings-on as it might result in me missing a critical change in my kid. That was not on my agenda. Rosa put her hand on her sister's shoulder as she recovered from the initial shock, and stood up. Carefully Rosa updated her on what was happening, and she began to relax. She hugged her parents as they stood inconspicuously in the background and Rosa broached the matter of going home. *Thank you, Rosa, for saving me from asking you guys to leave,* I thought.

"We've had enough stress for today, Tabitha," she said, "and we all agree that we will go home now, as it is very late. We'll be back in the morning." *Excellent.*

"I can imagine you are all worn out, Rosa," I paused. "I'll let you know if anything happens Rosa. I've got your phone number."

I checked the contact number with her again. *Yep, I had it.* And, as the family got ready to leave, they squeezed Homero on the arm, his mom rubbed his legs and then kissed his hand, and then they trouped out. It would take them almost two hours to get home, and it was almost midnight now. Rosa made a final check that the contact number was correct, and having no cell phones between them, she left saying, "I'll call you when we get home."

Homero's mom cried softly as she left. This time she was supported by Rosa and Isabella, as she stumbled out of the door, leaning heavily on them. Homero's dad brought up the rear, walking slowly behind them along with Rosa's friend and Isabella's fiancé, who had been waiting outside the room for a while. It was a sad little procession. It had been a very long day for them all.

With the space cleared, I turned back to the monitors, orders, and documentation. It would be peaceful without the family to divert my attention. I was busy enough transfusing blood products, watching vital signs, documenting, drawing labs and doing whatever appeared next on the list of orders.

However, within half an hour of the family leaving, Homero's condition worsened considerably. His blood pressure began to fall dramatically, and I called for Kirk.

"I don't like the look of what's going on…get a dopamine drip going," he said as he wrote the order. "I'm calling Dr. L."

Ding-dong.

"Bernie. Please come to Room 14, Bernie."

In seconds Bernie re-appeared, He was dragging the Code Cart from 20-feet down the hall, and parked it outside Room 14 —just in case.

"Can you check this dopamine order with me and get it running pronto?" I asked. "Things aren't going too well."

Bernie sprang into action, and within minutes the dopamine was running. He had dropped off three pediatric infusion pumps earlier in the shift —in case we needed them, and the Code Sheet that the day nurse had printed up when she admitted him stated that we would give him adult doses of all the drugs if he coded, because of his size. We were ready for anything. Glad that the cart was nearby, I tried to ignore it stationed outside the door. I heard the tail end of Kirk's conversation with the Intensivist. "Thanks, I appreciate you coming in," he said, as he hung up the phone.

Within seconds Homero's heart stopped. I pushed the Code Blue Alarm, and in an instant the team materialized. We heaved Homero onto his side and shoved the backboard under him in time for Bernie to start compressions. We hooked Homero up to the defibrillator and kept a practiced, rapid rate of compressions going. He was still on the ventilator. Support staff quickly drew up adult-sized volumes of Code drugs, and I took charge of documenting the Code: saturations, blood draws, compressions...drugs administered, blood pressure (none), more drugs, more compressions. The RT manning the ventilator disconnected Homero from it, and started bagging him in conjunction with Bernie's compressions.

Kirk handled the Code with aplomb from the start. Labeled Code meds lay ready on top of the cart, with an abundance of flushes as Sophia, the runner, took control of giving the meds. Kai dropped by. He was extra tall, and volunteered to take turns with Bernie on the cardiac compressions, and another RT came in to help Florence bag.

"Okay guys...let's stop and check for a pulse," Kirk ordered.

Glad for a short break, everyone stopped, and Bernie and Flo checked Homero's carotid and brachial pulses.

"Nothing."

"Flat-lining," someone else called –and I wrote it down.

"Proceed," Kirk called, and the Code continued. Relieved of compressions Bernie, as Charge Nurse, went to call the family. They would not be home yet, but he left a message asking them to call for an update. That was all he said.

When the Attending arrived to take over the Code, I called out what medications, blood products, and other fluids Homero had received intravenously and when they'd been given. As the first round of drugs had done nothing, everyone stood back, and the paddles were applied.

"Stand clear," called the nurse holding the paddles. "All clear."

Homero jumped with the shock from the paddles – but still flat-lined. Another Resident took over the cardiac compressions, but being short, she had to stand on a riser to get better leverage. Another PICU nurse joined Sophia in pushing medications and drawing labs. And so the Code continued.

"Hold it," the Attending called, and the staff checked for a heart rate. They defibrillated Homero two more times with increased power, but still without success. We gave four, full-rounds of drugs and different staff took turns with the compressions.

Nothing.

The RTs hand-bagged Homero, taking turns and occasionally attaching him to the ventilator. As the lab results came up on the screen, hope evaporated. It became more and more unlikely that Homero would ever come back.

More than an hour passed. The family returned Bernie's call when they got home and found his message. Bernie spoke with them —but did not give the whole story, and immediately they turned around and started the long journey back to the PICU.

And the Code continued. More medications, more blood gases, more shock treatment, more cardiac compressions —and no sign of life returning. Homero was clinically dead.

One and one-half hours into the Code, it was decided that the staff would continue the cardiac compressions and hand-bagging until Homero's family arrived —even though it was unlikely that Homero would ever respond.

Another 15 minutes passed. Bernie was doing cardiac compressions again, when the intercom crackled into life.

"They're here. I'm holding them for you," the secretary said from the front of the unit. They must have broken every speed-limit in an effort to get to IVCH.

Kai took the compressions over from Bernie, who went with the Attending to the front of the unit. The family was already in what we often referred to as the Grief Room. With Bernie at his side, the Attending gently told the family that Homero would not make it, and that it was our compressions, the ventilator, and the medications that were keeping him alive at the present time. The message was brief —and devastatingly final. Overwhelmed, they asked to see Homero.

While the Attending was talking with the family, it was all-hands-on-deck in Homero's room to clear the room of stuff, and staff. We removed unnecessary equipment and trash bags full to over-flowing of surplus dressings, cables, and tubings, intravenous bags and used equipment. We cleared away items strewn on the bed and floor, and calm returned in the nick of time.

Ding-dong. "They're on their way."

Homero's mother was the first to come in the room. She was weeping. Bernie spoke to the family as they entered, explaining what was happening and Kirk stood to the back of the room.

"Homero's still breathing," Bernie said, "and his heart is functioning with the compressions, but if they stop," he said, looking at Kai who was performing chest compressions, and Flo, who was bagging, "Homero will be dead. There's nothing else we can do."

Wake Up, Son

Bernie stopped talking. You could hear a pin drop. Homero's parents were in cataclysmic shock. Haltingly, Bernie started to speak again.

"We've given him all the medications we can ..." he said directing their gaze towards the defibrillator and the Code Cart, "and shocked him with the paddles." The room was silent. "I'm very sorry," he mumbled as he stepped over to stand beside me. I was sitting on a high stool, updating Homero's records with basically nothing.

Wordlessly, Homero's mom stood back, and let her husband come to Homero's left side, while Rosa went around Homero, to his right side. Kai, now standing on the lift, towered over everyone as he quietly continued cardiac compressions. However, suddenly Homero's dad reached under Kai's arms and started frantically pounding on Homero's chest with his fist. He was thumping Homero's chest at twice the speed of Kai's compressions. Kai moved over to give a little more space to Homero's dad and then Homero's dad started shouting at Homero.

"Wake up, Son ... wake up! Don't leave us...open your eyes...wake up, son," he yelled as he pounded his son's chest beneath Kai's long arms. It was Spanish, but I knew enough Spanish to make out what he was repeating. His voice got louder as tears rolled down his cheeks, and the pleadings continued. The room was silent except for the grief of the family. Isabella squeezed through and put one hand on Homero's leg and the other on her dad's shoulder. I imagined that she was telling her dad that it was no use, and that he should give up beating on Homero's chest —that it was too late.

I looked down at my documentation. There was little to write now. The monitors were off and, in essence, Homero was dead. A tear splattered onto the doctor's orders.

On Homero's right side, Rosa held up her mother. Tears rolled down their faces as they pled with Homero to come back to life, to keep playing soccer and not to leave them. Rosa's friend stood at the back of the room, almost against the wall, alone. Watching. Boxes of tissues made the rounds as Homero's family wiped their eyes, drying fountains of tears.

In a while, the pleadings lessened and Dr. L, the Intensivist, came in. He stepped forward and spoke to Rosa. His gentle voice showed no edge of impatience.

"Homero's dead, you know," he said. "We can't bring him back to life."

It was Homero's little, grebe mother who backed away first. It was over. Homero was dead. However, Homero's dad would not give up yet. He stood at Homero's side, pounding on his chest intermittently. It was futile, and eventually he stopped the pounding and the Attending gave the nod.

I sat unobtrusively in the corner and checked the time. Imperceptibly the compressions and hand-bagging ceased as the Attending moved quietly to Homero's side and listened to the silent chest. He then looked up at the family, saying, "I'm sorry. He's gone."

Homero was declared officially dead.

"03.58. Patient declared expired," I wrote. End of sentence. End of life.

The family stood at the bedside for a few minutes, and I edged slowly over to Rosa.

"If you can step outside for a short while, we will clear away more of the equipment so that you can spend time with Homero," I said. "I'm afraid we will have to leave the tube in his mouth, and some of the IVs in place –it's the law you know. I'm sorry."

Rosa passed the message on, and the family left for the Grief Room as we cleared Homero's room of the remaining IV pumps, Code Cart, and ventilator. We removed the backboard, capped the IV's and laid Homero's head on a soft pillow. Fresh sheets were draped over his body making him look as though he was sleeping peacefully, except the breathing tube pointed ominously towards the ceiling. It extended about eight inches upwards. Now, totally useless, it was a crude reminder of what had just happened. the situation. Last of all, we brought extra chairs into the room and more boxes of tissues, which we opened and placed on counters.

I left Room 14, pulling the curtains across the door. Someone had taped a small laminated bear to Homero's door and the hall windows, and a little later Homero's grieving family filed quietly back into his room. Isabella immediately lapsed into uncontrollable sobbing at the sight of her little brother. Her sobs, and the muffled sniffles of others, leaked out across the station. It was a sad reminder of tragedies that should never happen. Nothing would be the same again for another family.

After a while, I walked hesitantly towards the door. *Shall I go in now, or is it too soon? How would I feel if I were in their shoes? How much time would I want? A lifetime?*

Wake Up, Son

I turned around, and sat back at the station.

Fifteen minutes later, I drained the dregs of tea from my mug, and got up. *How about now?* The truth is they would never be ready. I pulled the door quietly back, and entered.

"Is there anything I can help you with?" I asked Rosa foolishly.

Obviously, there was nothing remotely helpful that I could do. The only thing they wanted, was for Homero to come back to life. If Jesus had been walking through the PedsICU today, this wouldn't have happened, and if it did, Jesus would have brought Homero back to life with just two words, "Homero, arise!" –just like He raised Jairus' daughter to life –and we'd all be out of a job!

"No, we're alright, thanks," Rosa half-smiled.

"Okay ... I'll be back in a little while. Let me know when you are ready."

I made my way back to the Nurses Station and sat down. Everything was quiet. This was a terrible night. *What if Homero was one of my sons? How would I deal with it? Thank God I can go home and hug my kids again.*

A while later, the door slid open, and I sprang off my chair, joining the family as they filed out of the room. I walked with them to the front of the unit.

"Yes, Homero's body will be going to the morgue ... It will be a coroner's case ... Do you know which funeral service you'll use? ... I'll call you in the morning with the numbers ... I'm so sorry."

I remained by the secretary's desk as the family left the floor. Strangely, this time it was Homero's mother who held up her husband. She led the way —and her family trailed behind her. What an amazing woman. Where did that strength come from?

The unit doors swished shut behind them. Another family, numb with sorrow and without hope, had left their child behind in the PICU. I slumped onto the counter. I was drained —and yet strangely warm inside. I had been privileged to care for Homero to the very end.

CHAPTER 7

Drawing the Short Straw

DEATH CAN BRING RELIEF. The inevitable has happened. It is over. But sadly, in the PICU, the pall of death is rarely wholly out of sight. It waits around the corner for another unsuspecting child. The list of causes of death is endless. All devasting deaths. From drowning, abuse, asthma, diabetes, infection, trauma, GSWs, heart disease, suicide, accidental ingestion of poisons, suffocation, fire —and still the list goes on. Each category represents little people who drew the short straw in life. Some were in the wrong place at the wrong time. Sitting on the sofa watching TV when the bullet came through the window, unable to stop their skateboard as it careened into a passing truck, or thrown from the family car because no one had insisted they wear a seatbelt. Maybe their parents were too young, or unwittingly negligent, abusive, or absent, when they needed them the most. Surely the kid didn't mean to kill themselves –or kill a friend. Maybe an innocent game took a wrong turn. Whatever it was, the result was the same. They made it through our doors, or didn't, but never went home.

Another life lost. Gone forever.

And then there are a special sub-group, a heart-breaking, unique, sub-group: the near-drowners, like. Ivan, Tiffany, Alan, Celine, Zach and little Tyler. They slipped silently into jacuzzies, a horse trough, a pool, a bath or simply tipped into a bucket when their mother's back was turned as she mopped the kitchen floor. Some were less than two years old. They made it through our doors —but going home? Maybe never to their own home. They might never graduate from kindergarten or play like regular kids in the sunshine. But birthdays. They would have those, at least some.

What nurse chooses to care for little kids that don't make it, and place them gently in their mother's arms when it is all over? PICU nurses do this with big hearts, gentle words and a prayer. Their mothers were there for their child in their final hours, but were missing, or distracted, at the time when they were most needed.

But Jacob's mom took us to a whole new level of indifference.

* * *

Fourteen years old and bald, Jacob had endured months of cancer treatment. Now, with us in Peds ICU, he spent most of his time lying on his left side, with his face away from the door. Was the left side his most comfortable side, or was he deliberately trying to remove himself from any reminder as to where he was, and why? Frequently Jacob requested medication to alleviate the pain in his bloated abdomen. But where was his mother?

"Jacob isn't doing well tonight," I said to her answering machine. "Please come and see him. He needs you."

Tonight was my second night with Jacob, and I had left a similar message with her the night before.

"Did she come today?" I asked Molly, as I got report that evening.

"What do you think?" Molly replied.

"No?"

"Right. His mom called at about ten this morning, and said she could not get a ride to the hospital. She lives 40 miles away, you know."

"Yes —but that is why we have Grainger House, Molly. Did you tell her that?"

"I sure did. But she wasn't interested."

Jacob's mother did not have time for him, as usual. She seemed to have other, more important things to do than sit at his bedside, love on him, hold his hand and be his advocate. Yes, she lived 40 miles away, and yes, she didn't have a car...but Jacob was dying, perhaps dying today.

"She said she would visit him on the weekend, when she could get a ride."

"But it's only Wednesday today!" I said incredulously. "He probably won't be here then. Did you tell her that?"

"I did all I could," Molly said. "She told me that he would be alright on his own. He was 14 years old, and not a baby. Jacob could wait."

But he absolutely couldn't wait.

I went in to access Jacob, and, in passing, told him that I had left a message on his home phone.

"Don't bother. She won't come," he growled.

Jacob knew his mother better than I did. He knew she didn't make him a priority in her life. She never had.

During the shift I offered Jacob pain medication as often as it was prescribed, unless he was asleep. In that case, when he awoke and asked for it —I gave it. I didn't care that he was getting a lot of medication for pain. It was ordered, and so what if he was getting addicted to it? He knew he was dying, and he was alone. In my estimation, his mental anguish alone warranted a dose of medication. I would have wanted to zone out if I was in such a deserted position, and in pain.

Like Jacob's other nurses, I didn't connect with him at a deep level. He had been disappointed, hurt and emotionally abused for too many years, and he knew what his future held. He wanted the agonizing physical and emotional pain that he had been in for so long, to stop.

That night Jacob died peacefully in his sleep. His face was still turned away from the door towards the wall. Alone, he slipped into death. There were no heroics, because he was a No Code. Finally, he was at peace. But I wasn't. I was angry that Jacob's end was so lonely, even if, at that time, he was actually pain-free. The sad end to a beautiful life was absolutely unacceptable. Jacob had drawn a very short straw.

* * *

A single loss of life on the PedsICU affects all the staff in one way or another. It is painful —but it happens. We expect a death from time to time. But, after a child dies, nurses check their patients' status a little more diligently. They do not want to experience the horror of another death soon, but occasionally it happens, again.

Multiple deaths in quick succession are devastating. Paranoia sneaks in. What went wrong? Why? What could we have done differently? What didn't we see? Perhaps I will call in sick —I can't face the possibility of another death.

Once, in three days, we lost three children!

Such a terrible happening was catastrophic for the whole unit, even though there is always an outside chance it could happen again in a large PedsICU, in a Tertiary Level Trauma Center. While nurses consciously, and subconsciously, deal with their own fears and a loss, they need to care for their patients for the shift in a positive, up-beat manner, hoping that they are on top of their game.

Drawing the Short Straw

* * *

The first of the three children was diagnosed with advanced meningococcal meningitis, always a challenging diagnosis. This put the staff immediately on high alert. In such cases, the loss of precious minutes can mean the difference between recovery (with some likely complications), and death.

Ham, short for Hammerstein, was ten years old and had been well until two days before he was admitted. For two days he had felt generally unwell. Then, after school on that particular day, his parents took him to their local hospital's ER with an aggressive rash.

Our Transport Team hot-loaded him from the desert community hospital, and brought him by air to the PedsICU. As the gurney sailed past my room, through the unit towards Station Four, I saw the Team performing chest compressions while standing on the gurney's lower rails, bagging him and pushing meds. Minutes before landing he had coded. Everyone was already wearing gowns, masks, and gloves and their efforts weren't in vain. In his room, they got him back in a short while and stabilized him —until he coded two hours later.

He never came back that time.

Ham's family arrived on the floor after he had passed away. It had taken them more than three hours to get to the PICU. They were too late. That unavoidable delay exacerbated the multitude of tough questions that began to race through their minds.

Why hadn't they acted sooner? Should the school have done something earlier? What could have been done differently? Was it their fault Ham died? *Why* did Ham die? Should they take IVCH to court about whatever happened? What was God doing when Ham died? Does God really exist?

Over the days and weeks ahead, their lives would be plagued by hundreds of questions, many of which had no good answer. It was a futile exercise. Ham was gone.

* * *

The next day, it was Matthew. He was an 11-monther who had been admitted two days earlier. He died from multi-system failure due to sepsis. He had three older sisters.

The brevity of his stay again made it difficult for the PICU nurses to develop a strong, supportive relationship with his parents. The two-plus days were filled with crises. His parents rode an emotional roller coaster, holding out for a miracle when Matthew was transferred into the PICU. But then, when his condition took a nose-dive, their despair and anxiety soared out of sight. Our doctors could not perform the miracle they had hoped for, and Matthew became another statistic for the infant mortality tables.

This second death, the second in two days, made the PICU staff nervous. We knew that we received critically ill kids from a very large catchment area, but might deaths actually come in threes?

"It's happened before," someone had said, adding "but that was before we had highly sophisticated medical treatments and advanced technology."

And the situation passed. But, the next evening, when waiting for the shift to start, Carissa glibly said, "Oh, they always run in threes!"

This riled me, but I should not have responded.

"Will you shush, Carissa?" I said. "Do you want to bring another death on us? Aren't two dead kids in two days enough?"

Number three was about to happen.

* * *

After only one day in the PedsICU, Kylie, a 16-month-old toddler died that night from either a non-accidental trauma incident or from SIDS, Sudden Infant Death Syndrome. She would be a Coroner's Case as the exact cause of death was unknown.

Again, none of the staff built a close, supportive relationship with Kylie's parents over such a short time. Possibly the parents were perpetrators of a crime but one couldn't assume anything. They were, perhaps, grieving parents, tragically losing their child to SIDS, something that no one wished on any parent.

The social work reports and police investigations added to the stress of caring for Kylie, making an exacting and hectic shift the more so. Our Intensivists and their team of physicians only wanted to see Kylie turn the corner and get better. But she didn't.

Although very occasionally deaths come in threes, usually not over three days, but in close succession, PedsICU nurses hope —and expect, that the next patient admitted to the floor will be a success story. We expect the child will be transferred to the Step-down ICU and then to a basic floor before going home to a loving family where they will enjoy a long, happy, healthy life because we were there when they needed us the most —and the PedsICU Team were the best! That's why we worked here.

* * *

A few weeks had passed since those three devastating deaths had occurred, and the staff had recovered. Debriefing sessions and the Spiritual Support Counselors helped with the staff's recovery, and many kids had been admitted, treated and transferred to the Step-down unit, before going home.

One afternoon Carrie admitted Anya to the PICU. Anya was 2 ½ weeks old. At first glance Carrie knew Anya was very ill, and she began to feel that rock-bottom, demon-in-the-chest feeling. The feeling of another impending death.

Young parents, living a distance from their own parents or other family members, miss the support provided by loving, experienced, mature people who have already seen a bit of life, which close-knit families used to provide. Consequently, as young adults, separated from family, they can miss the subtle signs of deteriorating health in a young baby. This delay can lose them valuable time in getting medical treatment if it's needed. Other young parents, who are on the neurotic end of the spectrum, rush to call their pediatrician's office —or their parents, at any little whimper, alteration in skin color, regurgitation, or loose stool.

Anya's parents did not fall into either of these categories. Young and astute, with excellent observation skills, they realized that something was wrong with Anya. However, having no health insurance, they delayed consulting a pediatrician and hoped their presumptions were imaginary. Eventually however, they took Anya to the nearest Emergency Room.

"She's not waking up…she only takes an ounce, if we are lucky…there must be something wrong…we think she is dying," they told the ER nurse. *Rather an exaggeration surely? A little dramatic?* But the distraught parents were right. Something was wrong. But dying? Anya was only two weeks old.

The ER staff realized that Anya was profoundly weak, practically too weak to breathe, so they intubated her almost immediately, thus protecting her airway. The first of many labs were drawn, and a peripheral IV was started to hydrate her. The ER doc called our Attending and the Transport Team was dispatched immediately. Anya was air-lifted to Inland Valley, directly to the PICU.

She arrived on the floor, strapped on the gurney. She was a tiny bundle of baby. Her cute little porcelain face peeked out of the blankets which were snuggly wrapped around her face, making her look like a tiny, beautiful, matryoshka doll. Carrie carefully unwrapped Anya and moved her gently to the baby scales as the RT bagged her, keeping a watchful eye on the ET-tube. Un-covered, Anya looked pale and wasted.

"Two-point-four-six kilos," Carrie announced to Carlos, the relief Charge Nurse assisting with the admission. Carlos entered the weight, put a new-born sized diaper on Anya and propped her up in the bassinet in the middle of the huge room. He covered her with a soft blanket and attached the leads to the overhanging screen. As Carrie got report from the Transport Nurse, Carlos sorted the IV pumps and extra equipment. The RT secured the ET-tube to the ventilator and after getting report, Carrie took Anya's vital signs and recorded them, assessed her, and re-wrapped her. The rectal thermometer read 101.8 ° F. Anya was a little febrile, but Carrie put it down to the fact that perhaps Anya had been wrapped too snugly for the flight.

The movement of the last few hours had distressed Anya and she cried, but without a sound as she was intubated. Her little eyes squeezed out tiny tears. She was piteous.

"I'll give her more sedation now, if you wish," the Transport Nurse volunteered. "The flight went well, but it was tough on her."

"Thanks. Anya will appreciate that —and so will I," Carrie said. "She's going to be busy for a while and I don't want her to suffer."

"She's been feeding poorly since coming home from the hospital," the Transport Nurse went on. "Her parents noticed quickly that she was weak, and they were worried — but did nothing. They're first-time parents, and don't look more than teenagers themselves. They didn't want to panic."

Carrie glanced down the Transport Physician's new orders: different IV fluids, central line placement, start pressors to maintain her blood pressure (if necessary), rectal Tylenol® for a fever, a broad-spectrum IV antibiotic to stop infection before it started, and diagnostics —a slew of labs, full body x-rays including an abdominal CT, MRI of the head and trunk, and more. As Anya started going through the tests, her parents arrived. They were shocked.

"Hi, I'm Carrie," Carrie said as they came into the room. "I'm Anya's nurse today." They nodded and smiled as they looked around the room. "This must be very distressing for your both," Carrie continued. "I'm sorry…Anya's in the right place…We're doing the best we can for her." Carrie watched them as she babbled on. "We are saving Anya's energy by breathing for her with this machine," she said, pointing towards the ventilator, "and giving her medications to keep her comfortable."

Anya's parents, Stephie and Alan, nodded their heads, trying to make sense of everything Carrie said. They were young and appeared petrified. They stood beside the bassinet with their arms around each other, watching Anya breathe in time with the ventilator.

Anya had been a planned pregnancy, everything had gone well, and they were thrilled when she was born a few days early, just two weeks ago. Like other excited, new parents, they dreamed of their little daughter's future. "Look at her tiny fingers…and toes…and her lips. They are like little petals," Stephie had said as she admired their daughter for the very first time.

Was it only two weeks since they first saw her, kissed her little lips, and held her tenderly in their arms? She was theirs —all theirs. They dreamed of her future, of her first smile and of her sitting up, getting her first tooth, crawling, walking and saying her first words. They planned to write down everything about her in the "Baby's Firsts" book. Stephie had filled only two pages in Anya's book. There were 38-pages still to go. There were pages for Anya's favorite toys, her first words, her first friends and for five birthdays.

How excited they were anticipating her starting kindergarten, having friends over to play, and for sleepovers. Anya would keep making memories for them. There would be her first formal, her high school graduation (and maybe even college) and then finally, meeting the man of her dreams, and marrying him. After that, she would have her own children. But for now, in their eyes —no one was more beautiful than their sweet little Anya.

A day passed and the tests were checked off one by one. The results started to roll in, and reality started to change for Anya's parents. Life looked bleak. Our Intensivist consulted pediatricians in other specialties, who then ordered more diagnostic tests. Soon, the uncertainty of everything became too much for them, and Stephie broke down in tears often.

"Anya's becoming an object for medical science," she protested between sobs. "I don't think I can sign off on one more test."

The anxiety was ripping her heart out, even though both Stephie and Alan knew that it was necessary for the medical team to find the exact cause of Anya's illness. They needed a diagnosis. Then it would be treated, and the tide would turn for them. Anya would get better. But, at first, nothing gave them hope.

More time passed. Anya was stable, but still on the ventilator. The medical team decided that some of the diagnoses did not match Anya's weak condition, but eventually, the Pediatric Neurosurgeons unraveled the mystery —and it could not have been worse.

"I'm sorry," the young surgeon said as he stood beside the little crib with Anya's chart in his hands. "The good news is that we know what the problem is," he said flatly. Stephie and Alan dared to hope again. A diagnosis at last. But then he continued, "The bad news is that Anya has an extensive tumor encapsulating her spinal column, and we can do nothing for her. Anya has terminal cancer."

Stephie's knees buckled as she collapsed into a chair.

"Terminal?" Alan mumbled. "But she's only three weeks old," he stammered.

After extensive discussions with the Pediatric Neurosurgeons and the PICU Intensivist and his team, Stephie and Alan were satisfied with the facts. They wanted Anya's life to be as pain-free as possible. There was nothing anyone could say to remove the pain they felt in their hearts, but over the next hours, Stephie and Alan chose for Anya to receive comfort measures only. No heroics. No more unnecessary tests. No sticks. No more diagnostics. Nothing.

PICU nurses have big hearts which they hide carefully under a layer of professionalism. We wish never to witness parents with only a hand of bad cards to play. We don't want parents to have only a selection of undesirable, ugly options from which to choose. Unfortunately, though, that was Anya's parent's lot, and such a horrible situation was painful for the staff to see.

Pink, laminated little bears were stuck to the glass windows surrounding Anya's room, and we drew the curtains. The unit's Social Worker and Chaplain were on hand to help Anya's parents with specific questions regarding funeral arrangements and burial, and the Chaplain gave them spiritual support when they asked for her. Vital signs were no longer vital, and the multitude of tasks that usually keep a PICU nurse busy, were minimized.

When Stephie and Alan heard that Anya wouldn't make it, they had to decide who they wanted to visit Anya. It was important for their nurse to make this terrible situation as painless as possible, and to accommodate all their wishes.

I was Anya's nurse on her final day. Anya was my only patient, so I was available to the family for anything. I stayed at the Nurses Station and assisted my colleagues when not required in Anya's room. Grandparents, aunts, neighbors and a few friends from Stephie and Alan's church filed slowly in and out of Anya's room. They prayed, hugged each other and whispered together until the Attending quietly walked into the room.

"Do you have any further questions for me?" he asked.

He looked little more than a school kid himself, appearing no older than Stephie and Alan, but his credentials showed years of experience. Married, but without children, he could only imagine the grief these young parents were experiencing. The Attending bent down beside Stephie and put his hand gently on her shoulder.

"Is there anything I can do for you?" He paused and dabbed his eyes. "I am so sorry," he said.

They could see he was very distressed, but they also knew why he was there. They knew there was nothing he could do for Anya.

He nodded at me. I turned off the monitor alarms and removed the leads from Anya as the RT turned off the ventilator alarms. Then I gently wrapped Anya in a blanket, and for the second time in less than four weeks, Anya's nurse presented her to Stephie to hold. This time though, Stephie was weeping.

I stepped outside, leaving Stephie and Alan gently holding Anya. Stephie's mom stood nearby, trying to keep herself together. She was distressed at witnessing her daughter's inexpressible pain, and for a few minutes Anya hung to the thread that was life. But as Stephie held her close, she died peacefully, free of pain.

If only sorrow could be wiped away with the ease with which the equipment was removed from Anya's room, but it can't. A potentially beautiful life had been snuffed out. Gone. This loss made me, the nurse who supposedly was as "tough as nails," cry.

Anya's straw was tragically short.

Drawing the Short Straw

* * *

It is very unusual for a baby to be born with cancer, but there were other little kids we saw who were a bit older, who struggled a little longer —and yet did not make it. They were caught tightly in the web of cancer: Julie Anne —and then Elizabeth, Bertie and little Davy. And the list still goes on behind those closed doors.

At times, the medical and nursing staff request a family consultation with the Medical Ethics Team during the extended care of such a critically ill, or dying patient. An ethics consultation brings together the full staff caring for the child, plus the unit's Social Worker and other support staff. The Medical Ethicist, usually a professor from the University, is the lynch-pin for the discussion. With the whole family present, they lay bare the clinical situation and the ethical dilemma facing everyone. The meeting helps the family understand more completely their options, and the decisions they are making for end-of-life care, if that is to be the case. It is vital that the family, if it has the time, has the opportunity to explore every avenue of treatment, and the probable outcomes before they make a decision that would result in withdrawing medical treatment from their child. After the child's death, recalling that meeting often provides comfort and an understanding of what happened, helping them to come to terms with their choices.

But the story doesn't end here for our kids' families. PICU nurses know that brighter days will dawn for Stephie and Alan, and for the hundreds of other grieving parents. They *will* smile again. The storm clouds of death *will* lift, and happiness *will* once again filter into their lives. PICU nurses know that. They've seen it happen.

During the grieving process, some parents return to thank the PedsICU Team for being there for them. They tell us of their struggles through the dark, empty months of pain and loss which eventually, gradually, lose their agonizing edge and turn into happier times, with lasting, sweet memories. Families reconcile their loss in the best possible way for them, and carry on life without their child.

I knew it would eventually happen for Anya's parents –at some time, but for now, they would endure the pain and emptiness that only the death of a child brings.

* * *

Sleep came slowly that night as my mind wandered through the last few hours of Anya's life and unanswerable questions. Did I do everything I could for Stephie and Alan? Could I have made Anya's death any less painful for them? Did I give them enough time alone with Anya after her death, or did I rush them so that I could cross my final "T" and dot my final "I"? Would Stephie and Alan's marriage survive this horrendous loss, or would it end up like so many marriages after the death of a child –in the divorce courts?

How I hoped that sharing a loss for which neither of them was to blame, would strengthen their relationship. I drifted to sleep aware of the honor that I'd had to be there for them through the worst hours of their lives.

It would get better for them one day.

I hope to meet Stephie and Alan in heaven with a cute little girl holding their hands. A smiling Stephie will say to me, "You remember her, don't you Tabitha?" And with my now-perfect memory, I will say, "I sure do, Stephie. This must be Anya. I remember Anya."

The Bible promises that heaven will be a place where all tears will be wiped away forever, and where family reunions will last for eternity —and I believe that.

CHAPTER 8

Nathan[1]

IT WAS 2.30 PM IN LATE SPRING, when the phone rang and I heard Mark's familiar, gruff voice at the end of the line. "Tabitha, can you come in now, pleeease? We have a transport arriving and no nurse."

I must be psychic. Planning on an early call and getting it? *Wahoo! But first, let him suffer!*

---

[1] Nathan is the real name of the child on which this chapter is based. Used by request.

"Well, Mark … I didn't sleep well last night … and I have four nights to go…"

"Pleeease come in Tabitha. We neeeed you."

"Okay, Mark. I was teasing –I'll be on my way. I was hoping you'd call. I need the money." *Why does anyone work if not for money?* Immediately swinging into accelerated action, I was in the PedsICU in less than 30 minutes. The unit was quietly buzzing. Corinne looked up, as I peered into her office.

"Room 13," she said without waiting for the question. "A 9-year-old. Multiple trauma." Corinne checked her report sheet and traced her finger down the listings to Room 13. "He was intubated in the field: leg fracture and abdominal injuries. He's in OR now. He's in critical condition, and his name is Nathan." I waited for more details. "That's all I know, Tabitha. Good luck."

Both of the nurses at Station Three had two patients. They were comfortably busy. They wouldn't be able to help me.

Hardly had I gotten the room ready than John, the RT, pushed a ventilator into the room. Close behind came Nathan. He was expertly maneuvered on a gurney by a team of four. An external fixator stuck out of either side of his fractured leg like pistons, and multiple IVs dangled from poles as the entourage passed down the hall. An RT clung to Nathan's side bagging him. *Whoosh...whoosh...whoosh.*

The nurse to the left of Nathan's head slapped the metal plate on the wall and the doors swung wide open. Hanging a right, the gurney glided through the doors and into Station Three. It swept past the first three rooms to Room 12 and, as though in a perfectly choreographed dance routine, the gurney went into reverse and backed into Room 13 head first, halting next to the bed. No one said a word. The crew expertly moved Nathan onto the scales as staff held every moveable bag, tubing, and blanket aloft, to get an accurate weight. With learned expertise, they lowered him onto the bed, rolled him to his right side off the weighing-cradle, and then from side to side to get the cradle out. Lying him on his back, we hauled him up the bed on a count of three and replaced the leads from the portable monitor with the overhead cable leads. Finally, the RT stopped bagging Nathan as he attached the new kid on the station to the ventilator. Nathan had arrived. Everything had gone like clockwork.

Like a freight train, the Recovery Room Nurse rattled through the report. Length of surgery, vital signs, input, output, medications. I scribbled to keep up with her. In short, Nathan had a fractured pelvis, a fractured left clavicle, a fractured right femur, a ruptured bladder, cuts and bruises, and abdominal injuries. That's all.

"It was a bad accident," the Recovery Room nurse said. "His dad's been admitted elsewhere. He's in a bad way, and Nathan is lucky to be alive. Nathan's brother is down the hall —but he'll be home soon," she added as she concluded her report. At least something was going well for Nathan's brother!

I didn't believe in luck, good or bad. I believed that every kid (and adult) had a Guardian Angel and that God allowed bad things to happen to good people because He was omniscient, He knew everything. At least that is how I rationalized my sister's death years ago, and I had found support for my faith in the Bible.

MVA admissions were usually associated with carelessness on someone's part. Kids not wearing seatbelts, a worn tire which is not recognized as a risk before it is too late, or drivers on the wrong side of the road. Drivers disregarding speed limits, intoxicated or high on drugs, failing to check for traffic carefully, young drivers and distracted drivers —they were all on the roads and putting innocent peoples' lives at risk every day. To me, driving was a serious business, and yet I still did foolish things behind the wheel at times. But are MVAs actually bad luck, or the result of poor choices —or both?

"I'll leave his papers with the secretary," the nurse said as she slipped the post-op documents into the chart. "Any questions?" I stared at her, and said nothing. "Well…I'm going. Good luck."

That was my second "good luck" of the day!

The accident had happened on a major highway that traverses the California desert, not far from the small community where Nathan lived with his mom, his brother, and his half-siblings. His maternal grandmother, Vera[2], lived up the street from them. In just seconds a family's life had changed. Devoted to Nathan, Grandma Vera later became an almost permanent fixture in our unit, and a vital link in Nathan's recovery.

Nathan was in critical condition, and the first challenge facing me over the next 16-hours was to get him stabilized —and to keep him stable. An A-line made monitoring his vital signs accurate and easy to monitor and the many medications he needed were delivered right to Nathan's room at first. Good IV access was important, and soon, with a central line in place, that problem was solved.

---

[2] Vera is Nathan's grandmother's real name. Used by request.

Documentation became a formidable task, but Nathan looked good and the night was young —so young that the rest of the night staff hadn't arrived yet.

Oblivious to the busyness of his room, Nathan slept, chemically sedated and free of pain. I set the alarms to warn me of a falling blood pressure or excessively high pressure, a dangerously slow or fast heart rate. But my single pair of hands was woefully inadequate for the multiple orders that kept piling up as "STAT" and "ASAP" orders. These took priority over documentation, the bane of every nurse's life.

In time Nathan's family began to course through the room in ones and twos, diverting my attention from matters on hand. Dismayed by Nathan's condition, and overwhelmed by the intense atmosphere of the PedsICU, some family members burst into tears when they first saw him, while others put on a brave face, expressing hope for his recovery, and appreciation for his care. And, as I expected, the questions came, "How is he doing?... What is his temperature? ... Can he hear me? ... Can I touch him? ... Will he get well? ... When will he be home? ... Have you ever looked after a kid like this before? ... What are the visiting hours? ... Who's his doctor? ..."

Nathan

Nathan's family was desperate for information but also blind-sided by his condition. My factual responses and the vague answers regarding his recovery, satisfied them for the present time.

"Nathan is very critical... *Does he look well to you?* His recovery will be slow... *Slow, as in more than a couple of days, and less than a year.* You will be able to talk to his doctors in the morning... *But they will give you the same, less-than-specific answers, because no physician is going to assure you that Nathan will recover and be as good as new.* They'll answer your questions in more detail..." *Can I please have space to catch up with everything, before I am submerged by my growing to-do list?*

Over the weeks, Nathan's visitors repeatedly traveled many miles from their desert community, and elsewhere, to visit him, and I grew to appreciate them more and understand the family dynamics. That's what happens when you look after a kid for a while —their family becomes your extended family. In turn, they became accustomed to the intense atmosphere of the PedsICU, to the sounds of the monitors and ventilators, the various alarms and endless hurry of the floor. The once unfamiliar, scary unit becomes, not by choice, a second home to them with faces they recognize, routines they know and medical procedures that become mundane.

Worn out from that first extended shift, I slept well the next day and returned for a 12-hour stint the next evening. I dealt with more physicians' orders, changing infusion solutions and troubleshooting pumps, transfusing blood products, administering medications, drawing labs, maintaining optimal sedation levels, lavaging Nathan's bladder, and performing extensive dressing changes.

Shifts flew by like greased lightning, and they became the norm for me and the other nurses who cared for Nathan. Those activities, coupled with the requisite documentation of vital signs and narrative comment, made each shift exacting and tiring, and, as the days passed, the shift reports became increasingly complex and longer.

An emergency head CT showed increasing pressure in Nathan's brain, so a bolt was placed in it to monitor its internal pressure and therefore direct the treatment ordered by the Pediatric Neurosurgeons. Nathan's kidneys were barely functioning after such a horrific trauma, so a large intravenous catheter was placed in his groin. It would be used for acute hemodialysis. The Pediatric Nephrologist and her team wrote those orders. A growing group of physicians, nurses, and techs cared for Nathan, and on his third day, the Pediatric General Surgeons performed the first of many abdominal surgeries.

Nathan

At last, after four nights of rigorous work and stressful challenges, I had two blissful nights off. But, by that fifth morning I had decided that I wanted to care for Nathan over the long-haul, even though I had no clue as to how long the long-haul would be.

"I want to primary Nathan," I announced to the Night Charge Nurse as I flopped down in a chair in her office.

The option to Primary a patient appeals to all PedsICU nurses at one time or another, but the decision isn't taken lightly. If a nurse primaries a kid, every time she is scheduled to work, she has to care for her kid, and that might include successive admissions too –especially if the kid has a chronic disease and becomes a frequent flyer.

"Is Monica working (or whoever the nurse might be)?" the kid's parent will ask as they come to the floor. "Monica is Alana's nurse, you know. She's her Primary Nurse. Is she here today?" So Alana gets her own nurse caring for her from the get-go on each admission. These kids are likely to experience decreased stress when they are re-admitted, and recover more quickly than if they had a different nurse for each admission. At some time, Alana will probably proudly say, with a big grin on her face, "Didn't you know, Monica's my nurse?" How special it makes a kid feel to have her very own nurse! And

Primarying also works well for the nurse and the patient's family, usually.

Primarying does have its downside though. Nurses coming on for two or three shifts in a row, don't want to take a primaried kid, as they know they will be bumped when the official Primary Nurse comes back from her time off —*no siree*. And it can be a huge commitment, unless a rift develops in the relationship between the family and the nurse, or the nurse becomes emotionally affected by her patient's care and the family's life, and feels no longer able to care for the patient in a professional capacity.

"It's like this," I explained to the Charge Nurse after she had filled in the application, "I like a challenge, and Nathan looks like a challenge-in-progress to me."

"You're right on that one," Anna agreed, "and this is only the first week. He'll be a heck-of-a-challenge for a very long time."

"Exactly," I interjected. "I think Nathan will keep me busy for a very, very long time."

Anna and I went back a long time. We lived near each other, went to the same church, and knew each other's kids well –and dogs! She was one of two night-shift Charge Nurses, but more importantly, she was a very good friend.

"And I like the older kids," I added, as though I had to persuade her further. "Big kids are much more fun than little kids in my opinion." Anna knew that too, of course. "I like working with kids Nathan's age, helping them overcome daunting challenges. I'm sure he'll have a few of those," I laughed. "He'll fit that bill to a tee! He'll be a great patient to primary, at least I hope so. I'm already going dizzy with everything that is going on with Nathan when I give report. Who knows what'll get lost in the process if he doesn't get a Primary Nurses soon?" *Had I convinced Anna yet?* "And, you know Anna," I said, as though I was flogging a dead horse, "his family is struggling with this accident, because more than one member of the family was hospitalized." I paused. "And they live so far away from here." I rolled on —just one more point to go. "Primarying will be helpful to both Nathan and his family –and I like them. What's more, I think they actually like me!"

She beamed at this improbability. No-nonsense Tabitha had friends? *Wahoo*. It was the clincher. Anna smiled. She knew me well enough to know that under my tough exterior there was hidden, somewhere, a tender heart. She signed the document. It was a done deal. I would Primary Nathan for however long it took. Hopefully, everyone would be a winner, especially Nathan.

Over the weeks, Nathan became a pediatric medical challenge to a growing contingent of physicians and caregivers, not just to me. Initially, we admitted Nathan as a trauma patient under the care of the Pediatric Orthopedic Surgeons, with the Pediatric Intensive Care Team consulting for fluids and ventilation. These teams were joined by Pediatric Neurosurgeons and Nephrologists and their teams, and slowly more physicians joined to further Nathan's recovery including the ENT surgeons, Pain Service, Child Psychiatry, Urology, Plastics, Occupational Therapy, Physical Therapy, Nutritional Services, Ostomy Specialists, the PICU Social Workers and the Discharge Planning Team for the desert community.

Occasionally kids have more than one Primary Nurse, so it was no surprise when, about a month after Nathan's admission, Bianca was approved to be Nathan's Primary Nurse on the day shift. That was good for Nathan, for she had a sweet personality that endeared her to all her patients (and her colleagues).

"This is just great," I bubbled when Bianca took over for the first time as Nathan's day shift, Primary Nurse. "You being there for rounds in the morning, and me being here at night, will prevent any screw-ups, well —reduce them at least. It annoys me that Nathan's treatment plan has been screwed up a few times already, despite everything. Having a day-shift Primary Nurse is going to be great for Nathan –and for me."

Bianca focused on Nathan's wounds that were healing slowly. At first his abdominal wound, leg, chest and smaller wound dressings took almost an hour to do and had to be changed three times a shift. That, with all the routine nursing care we needed to do, made it impossible for one nurse to keep up with everything, so helpers were enlisted to reduce the dressing time. As the weeks passed, Nathan's dressings needed to be changed only every eight hours – usually twice on the night shift, and once on the day shift.

"I am thankful that Nathan is out for the count when we do his dressings," I said to a fill-in nurse. "They are not a pretty sight. Make sure you medicate him adequately –he needs it."

They weren't a pretty sight, and Nathan had to be loaded with analgesics, in excess of his normal needs, to make the dressing changes even bearable.

The busy schedule of medications and nursing care did not deter Bianca from aggressively dogging Nathan's physicians, plying them with his needs and her concerns. Expertise in skin care was her forte, and she stocked his room with boxes of dressings and different types of tape and ointments.

As a nurse on an adult medical floor, Bianca had gathered a lot of valuable knowledge and skin-care nursing skills. These stood her in good stead when caring for Nathan's huge abdominal incision, as well as fistulae that leaked stool and urine. Bianca relentlessly highlighted Nathan's skin problems, looked for alternative treatments, and initiated consults with the Ostomy Nurse and Plastics in an endeavor to speed up healing, and minimize the painful dressing changes.

Her diligence paid off. In time Nathan began to heal, and when he was well enough to respond to us, Bianca's upbeat cheerfulness won his heart. She became his favorite nurse. Was it any wonder?

Two weeks after Bianca became Nathan's day-shift, Primary Nurse, I found myself reporting to Joanna. I thought nothing of it because Joanna had taken care of Nathan a few times before. She sipped her coffee in readiness for a busy shift. She had boys who were older than Nathan, and a don't-mess-with-me attitude. It was good for Nathan to have Joanna for a shift or two, I thought. She wouldn't let him beg-off on anything.

"Okay, Joanna… let's get the show on the road," I said to fill in time as she got her report sheet ready. "How many days will you be on? I think Bianca will be back in two or three days."

Joanna looked up. "Don't you know Tabitha?"

"Know what?"

"I'm primarying Nathan on the day shift with Bianca. We usually work opposite each other, and I signed up to primary Nathan before I took my days off."

"That's great," I chortled. I did the math. Six out of seven days Nathan would have a Primary Nurse caring for him on the day-shift. *Brilliant.*

Fast forward another 2-months and Kai, a Night Nurse who had covered many of the night shifts when I was off, officially signed up to be Nathan's fourth, Primary Nurse.

"So you finally made it official, did you, Kai?" I sparked good-naturedly when I next saw him in the Nurses Lounge before the shift began.

"Yes, I have," he said, grinning broadly. I waited for the reason for the broad grin. "Now I'll have an official reason not to work with you! Why didn't I think of that before?" He gave me a friendly shove. "And not only that —you are the "bumpee" tonight. Double-whammy for you!" he added triumphantly. *Darn it!* As this was an extra night for me, and Kai was scheduled *and* Nathan's other official Primary Nurse, I had to take another kid for a change.

"Well," I replied, "you'd better watch out Kai, because two can play at the same game!"

And I did.

Nathan now had a full complement of Primary Nurses –four nurses committed to caring for him, each bringing their distinctive personalities into play, building unique relationships with Nathan and Grandma Vera who sat beside his bed most of the day shifts, and into the early evening.

I was the oldest nurse on the team —as Kai frequently reminded me, with high school and college-age kids of my own. On quiet evenings, Grandma Vera and I chatted about the social injustices of the world, matters concerning our spiritual journeys and how not to make Christmas pudding. A Brit to the core, Christmas fare was often close to my heart –and stomach, as winter neared.

Nathan

My interest in a patient's psychological well-being, especially in Nathan's recovery, forced me to request Pediatric Psychiatry to become involved in Nathan's care. The 24-hour continuum of activity in PedsICU had taken its toll on Nathan. His sleep was interrupted frequently, making him vacillate between agitation and depression, and although we saw Nathan making good progress, the daily routines were lamentably tedious and painful, and Nathan couldn't see even the tiniest of light shining at the end of the tunnel. He'd lost track of the first few weeks of his admission because he was drugged up and intubated, but the waxing and waning of pain, the repetitiveness of being suctioned, turned, pulled up in bed, rolled from side to side, waking with inadequate pain medication on board, or enough to endure yet another treatment, took its toll.

A very challenging time occurred in Nathan's ninth week in PedsICU. He became extremely agitated during the dressing changes, so much so that the dressings took increasingly more time to do, instead of less time, owing to the interruptions he caused. After four nights in a row, I had had enough. I was drained.

"I can't do another shift," I complained to Joanna. "I don't think I have met a more difficult kid in my life."

That was probably an exaggeration, but the difficulties the other nurses and I were facing, were cumulative, and I was at the end of my rope.

"I understand," Joanna replied. *Really? Is it that bad on days?* "We're all struggling, especially after two shifts in a row."

"Oh…" I conceded reluctantly, "—and I'm at the end of four."

That did not impress Joanna.

"Why not see how you are when you come back on Tuesday?" *What a brilliant suggestion! Great plan. Put it off for a few days —but I'm signing off on him. I've had enough.* However, when I came back after three nights off, I decided not to sign off on Nathan. Joanna had been right after all. I'd give Nathan my best shot again.

It was not long after this upset that Nathan started to emerge from his mental and physical challenges. Perhaps the antidepressants began to kick in. Whatever it was, the crisis was over, and he began to work steadily towards recovery with his teams of physicians and nurses. That was a direct answer to prayer. *Praise God!*

* * *

Bianca was the sweetest, kindest nurse a kid could ask for. She hugged Nathan and laughed with him. She praised him and spoilt him. She scolded him when he was lazy, and she became excited when things went well. When setbacks occurred, she would not concede to failure, but encouraged Nathan to try again. When Grandma Vera was despondent, Bianca's effervescent optimism helped her to bounce back too, and Bianca's determined attitude maintained the momentum of the medical teams.

Joanna, on the other hand, was less buoyant, and did not allow Nathan to manipulate her as most kids would try to when things became difficult. Her determined attitude maintained the energy of his physical recovery, and she particularly encouraged him with respect to weaning him from the ventilator, in his tracheostomy care, and in encouraging him to use of a Passé Muir valve which enabled him to talk through his tracheostomy. At first, Nathan's weakened condition made this a significant challenge, but Joanna insisted that he follow through with the plan, develop stronger muscles for breathing, and not to rely on the ventilator.

"You can do it, Nathan. Just 10 more minutes," Joanna insisted when he felt he couldn't work a moment longer at breathing or talking. "You can do it!"

And Nathan did. Nathan began to talk again, even though he rested at night, using the ventilator for ever shorter periods of time until he was finally free of the vent. A tremendous accomplishment. Her insistence had paid off.

Kai was Nathan's friend. He was an acclaimed long-distance runner, and his own kids were a similar age to Nathan. Nathan liked Kai's laid back, friendly attitude and his interest in sports. He kept Nathan up-to-date on important matters like baseball scores, football season news, and athletics. Later on, as Nathan recovered, occasionally Kai came in specially to watch basketball on TV with Nathan. Much later, when Nathan could eat real food, pizza and basketball was a winning social event for both of them.

Surprisingly I was the one who connected Nathan with his favorite team, the Miami Dolphins. I, who knew nothing about Miami, and nothing about the Dolphins, organized a special visit for him. Somehow I got the wheels turning in the right direction, and made a memorable day for Nathan and Grandma Vera when team members came to visit him. What excitement! What a blast! To see Nathan so thrilled was enough payback for me.

* * *

Nathan

Nathan was not the usual PICU kid. He was a very long-term-boarder, staying more than four months on the unit, with a further two months of rehabilitation on a Basic Pediatric Unit, but by the time he went home, he was a walking, talking, eating miracle! His was a success story of great magnitude —and he knew it. No lives were lost in such a serious MVA –that was a miracle too.

After his discharge home, Grandma Vera and Nathan returned for frequent follow-up appointments and minor surgeries. Once, when visiting, Nathan flipped up his shirt to proudly show off a new, thin scar, instead of an ugly, jagged wound, and, despite still having a limp, he ran along the hallway to the front desk —not as fast as Kai, but then none of us could do that!

From time to time, "Nathan's at the front everybody. Come on down!" echoed over the intercom system, and a group of his nurses stopped what they were doing and went to Station One to check out his progress. He had won a special place in the PedsICU nurses' hearts and seeing Nathan walking, chatting and grinning from ear to ear, gave their hearts a bolus of hope and love, which required hugs all around!

Since Nathan's accident, his life changed. Nathan had met death and conquered it. He had been given the gift of life a second time, and his bright eyes and happy smile proved that the PICU is a hope-generating factory where miracles do happen.[3]

---

[3] At time of printing, Nathan is in good health and married. He and his wife have three children. He is a Certified Medical Assistant and has a business degree. (Included with permission)

GLOSSARY OF TERMS

abdominothoracic (CT): scan of the abdomen (stomach) and thorax (chest)

A-line: arterial line; a specialized line placed in an artery to constantly monitor a patient's heart rate, blood pressure and more, and to provide means to draw arterial blood gases and blood samples painlessly

AML: Acute Myelogenous Leukemia

analgesic: pain killer, pain medication

apneic spells: no breathing over a short period of time repeated occasionally

Attending: Abbreviation for Attending Physician; a PICU Attending is also known as a Pediatric Intensivist

bag, bagging: providing a patient with oxygenated breaths by hand, using a special mask and bag; usually performed by Respiratory Therapists, but also by competent nursing and medical staff

bolus: large amount of medicine or fluid given over a short period of time, usually on one or a few prescribed occasions

CCTV: Closed Circuit Television

central line: an intravenous access line that allows large amounts of fluids, or medications, to be given to a patient rapidly; usually has multiple access points in the line

cerebral cortices: (plural of cerebral cortex) the exterior of the cerebrum which is the most highly developed part of the human brain and is responsible for thinking, perceiving, producing and understanding language.

Code Cart: mobile unit containing all the equipment necessary to conduct a successful Code Blue

Code: (n) AKA: Code Blue; emergency where prescribed emergency life support measures must be initiated immediately; **coded:** (v) past tense of carrying out the process of a Code

Glossary of Terms

COPD: Chronic Obstructive Pulmonary Disease; serious lung conditions usually found in adults

cranium: skull

DNR: do not resuscitate; AKA "No Code"

ER: Emergency Room

ET-tube: endotracheal tube; a tube connecting a patient to a ventilator (respirator) that delivers oxygenated breaths to the patient. The plastic tube extends from the machine tubing, through the patient's mouth (usually) and into the lungs

extubated: removal of an endotracheal tube

°F: degrees Fahrenheit; scale used in USA for measuring body temperature;

fasciitis: inflammation of the fascia, connective tissue that attaches, stabilizes and encloses muscles and internal organs

febrile: feverish; a body temperature exceeding the normal of 37° C / 98.4°F

fistulae: (plural of fistula) abnormal passage from one epithelial site to another surface

Float: a Float (nurse) is a nurse working on a floor that is not her usual workplace; a Float maybe hired to work a variety of floors regularly; to float means to go to work on a floor different from the nurse's usual place of work

flushes: usually syringes filled with normal saline to move medications rapidly along an intravenous line

GLF: Ground Level Fall

G-tube: gastrostomy tube; tube to deliver medications and feedings directly into the stomach through a surgically created opening in the abdominal wall

hemoc: abbreviation for "Hematology and Oncology", Hemoc Unit

hemodialysis: a process of purifying the blood of a person whose kidneys are not working normally

hot-load: to pick up a patient rapidly, usually without turning off the helicopter engine (blades), implies real urgency

hyperbaric oxygen therapy: oxygen provided under pressure to tissues to promote healing within high pressure chambers

ingest: swallow

intubate: to place a breathing tube into the lungs through the mouth, or nose, in order to mechanically support breathing

lavage: wash-out; clean out with water or saline usually

Tertiary Level Trauma Center: hospital authorized to care for patients rated as most critical, Level 4 & 5

MVA: motor vehicle accident

NAT: Non-Accidental Trauma, trauma inflicted intentionally or without caution; child abuse

NICU: Neonatal Intensive Care Unit

No Code: resuscitation status where a parent, or the next of kin, have authorized no treatment should be provided should an emergency occur; the same as DNR

one-to-one: one nurse caring for one, high acuity patient, over a shift

OR: operating room

Ostomy Nurse: nurse specializing in ostomy care, skin care

peds: (pronounced "peeds") abbreviation for "pediatric"

Primary Nurse: a nurse who signs up to care for a specific child when the nurse is at work over one or many admissions

RT: Respiratory Therapist

sepsis: a toxic condition resulting from the spread of bacteria, or their toxins, from a focus of infection; septicemia: sepsis of the blood, a life-threatening condition if treatment is delayed or the infecting organism is extremely virulent or resistant to treatment; **septic:** condition of sepsis

sickler: an abbreviation denoting a child with Sickle Cell Anemia

somnolent: drowsy; somewhat unresponsive

Step-down: abbreviation for Step-Down Intensive Care Unit, a unit which provides less specialized care than an Intensive Care Unit but more than in a Basic Unit

stick: common term used to describe obtaining blood samples from patient through a needlestick

-stomy: suffix for a surgically created, artificial opening to the skin's surface such as colostomy or tracheostomy

Supe: (pronounced "soup"), Supervisor

urometer: a collection device used to measure urinary output via a urinary catheter

ventricular drain: a mechanism that allows cerebro-spinal fluid drain from inside the brain (the ventricles) to drain into a sterile collection unit and to minimize brain injury and brain tissue swelling

ABOUT THE AUTHOR

TABITHA B. C. ABEL lived a quiet life in the English countryside with her mother and sister Rebecca, who was 19-months her elder. Before her arrival, her father and mother had lived the life of the rich (and not famous) in India for 20 years, but when the marriage soured, Tabitha's mum returned to England where Tabitha was born. Her parents divorced when she was two, in the 1950s. Her mum was on her own with two young children and life wasn't easy. The three older children soon became adults and, receiving no financial support, her mother was left to fend for the youngest children –despite her birth-family's wealth and the comfortable life she had lived in when married.

Tabitha trained to become a nurse at King Edward VII Hospital in Windsor, Berkshire and married a pastor in her early twenties. After becoming a State Registered Nurse, she studied midwifery at Halifax General Hospital in Yorkshire, gained her certification and practiced midwifery for the next nine years as they moved to different locations in the north of England. They had three children who are now adults, and still very important to her life.

In the early 1970s, Rebecca, the sister with whom she had grown up, was killed by a drunk driver in Queens, New York while she was with a friend on Christmas break. That incident introduced Tabitha to death at close hand, and dealing with loss. Rebecca had a full scholarship for graduate studies at Andrews University in Berrien Springs, Michigan.

In the early 1980s, and again in the early 1990s, Tabitha and her first husband, a pastor, moved between the UK and the US for study. Those were busy years and uprooting their young family three times to cross The Pond, to live in very different cultures, was another kind of trauma.

About the Author

While in southern California, Tabitha worked at Loma Linda University Children's Hospital and the Medical Center, and studied at Loma Linda School of Public Health, eventually gaining a Master's degree in Health Promotion and a Doctoral degree in Public Health, Health Education. Later she earned a Master's degree in Nursing Education, from the University of Phoenix.

Tabitha was privileged to work with an amazing team of nurses, physicians and medical professionals who tolerated her quirkiness in the various roles she filled in PedsICU from bedside nurse, to relief Charge Nurse, to potluck planner and editor of the monthly news-sheet, *PICK-U PostIt* –and general agitator and encourager. Some of those people are still her friends, keeping track of each other on Facebook and through occasional face-to-face gatherings and sporting events. Life moved on with her caring for other kids, in other locations, over a long career in nursing.

Despite her busy life as a mother –and less-than-perfect wife, student, nurse, and university and college adjunct faculty member, Tabitha flourished under pressure and delighted in many friendships. In time, her children grew up to make lives of their own and Tabitha moved to Oregon and then to Washington state.

Divorce is rarely pretty, and brought a lot of regrets but now, married to her second husband, Gary, she faces problems of another kind, as we all do. She still relies on God to get her through challenges today and now, retired from teaching and nursing, she continues to participate in short and medium-term mission projects and remains a competitive runner and triathlete, a free-lance writer, musician, hiker and weekly blogger at Tabel Talk@TabithaBCAbel on Facebook where she talks about This and That from a Christian perspective.

The story of Jesus bringing the daughter of a synagogue leader back to life as recorded in the Bible in Mark 5 and Luke 8 is one of Tabitha's favorites. But Jesus didn't stop there. He, a Jewish man in an age when women and children held no position in the hierarchy of Judeo-Roman society, invited children to spend time with Him in the temple —much to the surprise of His disciples (Matthew 19:13-15, Mark 10: 13-16; Luke 18:15-17) and had some strong words for those who treated children unfairly (Matthew 18: 2-6; Mark 9:42; Luke 17:2). He also respected women (John 8:2-11; John 19:26,27; Matthew 9:20-22; Mark 5:25-34; Luke 8:43-48) and touched lepers, the untouchables of His day (Matthew 8:1-4; Mark 1:40-45; Luke 5:12-15). Jesus was remarkable and stood up to the religious and political leaders of His day, who were intolerant of the marginalized and hated dregs of society.

Tabitha wishes that the Great Physician would walk through every PedsICU and pediatric floor, and heal all the kids but God still uses humans to bring about miracle healings. And, as His hands, Tabitha does her part to stand up for kids and for those stigmatized by society, even against the religious, social and political leaders of her day if needs be.

Tabitha believes that the stories contained in *KIDS IN CRISIS: PICU Kids, Our Heroes* will open reader's eyes to a world that they may never enter and help readers to better understand what goes on behind those closed doors. The KIDS IN CRISIS trilogy has been written to provide readers with an educational, human-interest perspective on PICU kids and pediatric nursing. This memoir is expected to fill a void in the present medical literature about caring for critically ill children.